喚醒你的英文語感！

Get a Feel for English !

喚醒你的英文語感！

Get a Feel for English !

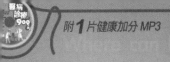

附 **1** 片健康加分 MP3

總編審：：王復國

作　者：：Lily Yang

醫病診療

900句典。

說不出病痛太離譜

Where can

Does anyone

lp is coming. Just

I'd like to see the GP

Where can

Does anyone kno

at does my blood pressure reading

mean?

Help is coming.

Just hang in

健康必備良方

☑運動

☑飲食均衡

☑900句典

貝塔語言出版

Beta Multimedia Publishing

Writer's Introduction

The last thing anyone wants while they're traveling is to get sick. Just imagine: you're in a foreign country, you may not speak the local language, and you probably have no idea where to get the help you need. "Overheard at the Hospital" provides you with useful sentences and important vocabulary. From finding a doctor, to answering questions, to making sure you get the medical care you need (and deserve), you'll find it all in this book.

With so many people traveling around the world these days, it's likely that some of them will fall ill during at least one of their travels. This handy book is a useful tool for anyone who goes overseas, be it students, businesspeople, or families on vacation. Some hospitals have started to employ translators, but this service isn't available everywhere. If you consider the panic that people feel in an emergency situation, or the inability to think clearly when they're in pain, it becomes clear that a basic knowledge of medical English is necessary for everyone who travels.

We hope you find this book both useful and interesting, and that you'll feel more secure on your next trip, knowing you're prepared for any situation.

Stay healthy, and good luck!
Lily Yang

作者序

外出旅行時，生病是大家最不願意碰到的事。想像一下：你人在異鄉，可能不會說當地的語言，或許也不曉得該上哪兒求援。《醫病診療 900 句典》提供讀者最實用的句子和最重要的字彙。從找醫生、回答問題，到取得（你應得到的）醫療資源，這些在本書中都找得到。

今日人們經常到世界各地旅行，或多或少會碰到生病的情形。這本隨身書非常實用，最適合到國外旅遊的人士，不論是學生、商場人士，還是舉家度假的人，全都用得上。有些醫院已經開始雇用翻譯人員，但是不見得每個地方都提供這種服務。如果你考量到人們在碰到緊急狀況時會慌張，或者是在身體疼痛時會沒辦法好好思考，那麼，對所有外出旅遊的人來說，具備和英語相關的基本醫療知識是相當必要的。

我們希望讀者會覺得這本書既實用又有趣，在你下一次出遊時會信心滿滿，因為你已經做好了充分準備，不論遇上任何狀況都不會驚慌。

祝福各位讀者健康、順心！

楊智媛 Lily Yang

CONTENTS

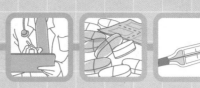

CONTENTS

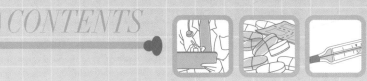

Part 5 診療第一步——和醫生對談

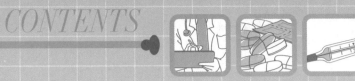

CONTENTS

Part 8 病人的問題與疑慮

Part 9 住院

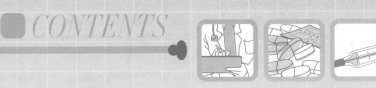

CONTENTS

Part **10** 意外和緊急事件

CONTENTS

Part 13 參考資訊

Part 1

好像生病了

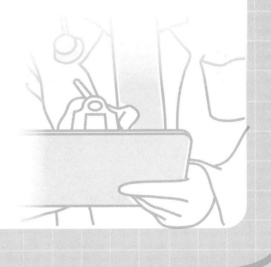

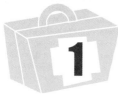

1 基本表達 I

☐ I don't feel very well.
我身體不舒服。

☐ I feel kind of sick.
我好像有點生病了。

☐ I may be coming down with[1] something.
我大概生病了。

☐ I feel really ill.[2]
我真的很不舒服。

☐ I'm a bit under the weather.[3]
我有一點不太對勁。

☐ I might have caught a bug.[4]
我可能感冒了。

Word List ▶ ▶ ▶

1 come down with *sth.* 得、染上（病）

2 ill [ɪl] *adj.* 生病的

3 under the weather 【口】不舒服

4 bug [bʌg] *n.* 病菌

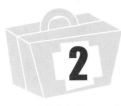

2 基本表達 II

☐ I think I'm going to puke.[1]
我覺得我快要吐了。

☐ Does my forehead[2] feel hot to you?
你摸摸看我的額頭是不是發燙？

☐ I think I have a cold.
我想我感冒了。

☐ My throat[3] hurts.
我喉嚨痛。

☐ My head is pounding.[4]
我頭在抽痛。

☐ Can you take my temperature?[5]
你可不可以幫我量一下體溫？

Word List ▶ ▶ ▶

1 puke [pjuk] *v.* 嘔吐
2 forehead [ˈfɔr͵hɛd] *n.* 額頭
3 throat [θrot] *n.* 喉嚨

4 pound [paʊnd] *v.* 鏗鏗地響；怦怦地跳
5 temperature [ˈtɛmprətʃɚ] *n.* 體溫

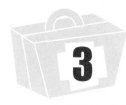

3 尋求協助

如果你知道自己生病了，可以用下列的句子尋求援助。

☐ Do you think I should see a doctor?
你覺得我應該去看醫生嗎？

☐ What do you think I should do?
你覺得我應該怎麼做？

☐ Can you help me find a doctor?
你可不可以幫我找醫生？

☐ Do you think it's serious?[1]
你覺得這很嚴重嗎？

☐ Where's the nearest pharmacy?[2]
最近的藥局在哪裡？

☐ Should I take any medicine, or should I just rest?[3]
我需要吃藥嗎？還是休息一下就好？

Word List ▶▶▶

1 serious [ˋsɪrɪəs] *adj.* 嚴重的
2 pharmacy [ˋfɑrməsɪ] *n.* 藥房

3 rest [rɛst] *n.* 休息

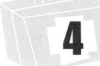

4 去診所，還是上醫院？

如果你只是有一點不舒服，去一般診所應該就可以了。如果病情嚴重，上醫院或許是必要的。

☐ **Do people here go to clinics[1] or hospitals[2] when they get sick?**
這裡的人生病時會去診所，還是上醫院？

☐ **Do I have to make an appointment[3] at the clinic?**
我去診所是不是必須預約？

☐ **Is it more expensive to go to a hospital?**
去醫院是不是比較貴？

☐ **Hospitals scare me. Is there a clinic nearby?**
醫院讓我感到害怕。這附近有診所嗎？

☐ **Will I have to wait long at a hospital?**
我上醫院會不會要等很久？

☐ **Do I really have to go to a hospital?**
我是不是真的必須去醫院？

Word List ▶▶▶

1 clinic [ˋklɪnɪk] *n.* 診所
2 hospital [ˋhɑspɪt!] *n.* 醫院

3 appointment [əˋpɔɪntmənt] *n.* 約定會面

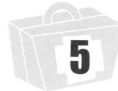

5 支付健康照護費用——如果你有保險

在台灣公司保的險

☐ I have travelers insurance[1] through China Trust in Taiwan. Here's my policy.[2]

我在台灣透過「中國信託」保了旅遊險。這是我的保單。

☐ Can I pay the deductible[3] with my credit card?

我可不可以用我的信用卡支付可扣除的金額？

☐ I'm going to need copies of all these forms for my insurance company in Taiwan.

我要把這些表格影印幾份給我在台灣的保險公司。

在國外的公司或機構保的險

☐ I'm covered by my university's student health insurance.

我唸的大學有幫我保學生險。

☐ My company is with Blue Cross. Here's my card.

我的公司保的是「藍十字」。這是我的保險卡。

☐ Is my treatment going to be completely covered by my HMO?[4]

「健康管理組織」是否會完全支付我的治療費用？

Word List ▶▶▶

1 insurance [ɪnˋʃʊrəns] *n.* 保險
2 policy [ˋpɑləsɪ] *n.* 保單

3 deductible [dɪˋdʌktəbl] *n.* (保險的自負額)
　可被扣除的金額
4 HMO = Health Maintenance Organization
　健康維護組織

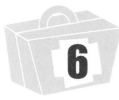

6 支付健康照護費用——如果你沒有保險

☐ I don't have insurance, but I really need to see a doctor.

我沒有保險，但是我真的需要看醫生。

☐ I don't know if I have enough money to pay for this.

我不知道我是否有足夠的錢支付這個。

☐ Is there a free clinic nearby?

這附近有免費的診所嗎？

☐ Does this hospital have some kind of payment plan?[1]

這家醫院有沒有提供什麼付款方案？

☐ Can you tell me how much it's going to cost ahead of time?
I don't have insurance.

你可不可以事先告訴我要支付多少費用？我沒有保險。

☐ I'd like to pay with cash, but I can only take $200 out of the
ATM.

我想付現金，但是提款機只能提領兩百元美金。

Word List ▶ ▶ ▶

1 payment plan [ˈpemənt ˌplæn] n. 付款方案

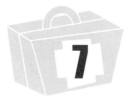
7 找好醫生

☐ **Do you know of a good doctor?**
你有沒有認識好的醫生？

☐ **Where can I find a list of doctors in the area?**
我在哪裡可以找到這一區的醫師名單？

☐ **Have you ever been to this doctor?**
你有沒有給這位醫生看過病？

☐ **Can anyone recommend¹ a good pediatrician²/ gynecologist³/ dentist?⁴**
有沒有人可以推薦一位好的小兒科醫生／婦產科醫生／牙醫？

☐ **Is it easy to obtain a doctor's credentials⁵ here?**
醫師執照在這裡容易取得嗎？

☐ **Does he / she answer all of your questions?**
他／她是否解答了你所有問題？

Word List ▶▶▶

1 recommend [ˌrɛkəˋmɛnd] v. 建議
2 pediatrician [ˌpidɪəˋtrɪʃən] n. 小兒科醫師
3 gynecologist [ˌgaɪnəˋkɑlədʒɪst] n. 婦科醫生
4 dentist [ˋdɛntɪst] n. 牙醫
5 credential [krɪˋdɛnʃəl] n. 證書

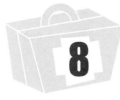

8 預約 I ——對方可能會這樣問

☐ Which doctor would you like to make an appointment with?

你想預約哪位醫生？

☐ Can I have your name / telephone number, please?

能不能請告訴我你的姓名／電話？

☐ Have you visited our clinic before?

你以前有沒有來過我們診所？

☐ What date / time are you looking at?

你想要哪一天／什麼時間看診？

☐ Your appointment is for Tuesday at 2:00 p.m.

你預約的時間是星期二下午兩點。

☐ Please remember to bring your medical records[1]/ insurance information[2]/ medication.[3]

請不要忘記攜帶你的病歷／保險單據／藥品。

Word List ▶▶▶

1 medical record [ˋmɛdɪklˋrɛkəd] n.
就醫紀錄

2 insurance information
[ɪnˋʃurəns, ɪnfəˋmeʃən] n. 保險資料

3 medication [.mɛdɪˋkeʃən] n. 藥物（治療）

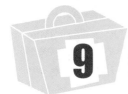

9 預約 II——你可以這樣回答

☐ I'd like to make an appointment to see Dr. Webber.
我想預約韋伯醫生的門診。

☐ Is Dr. Lee available[1] Thursday morning?
李醫生星期四上午有沒有空？

☐ Do you take morning / afternoon / evening appointments?
你們接不接受早上／下午／晚上的預約？

☐ Could you please give me directions[2] to the clinic / hospital?
可否請你告訴我去診所／醫院該怎麼走？

☐ How much does a basic consultation[3] cost?
初步診療的費用要多少錢？

☐ Do I need to register[4] at the front desk[5] when I arrive on Wednesday?
我星期三到的時候需不需要先到櫃檯掛號？

Word List ▶ ▶ ▶

1 available [ə`veləbl] *adj.* 有空的
2 direction [də`rɛkʃən] *n.* 指示
3 basic consultation [`besɪk͵kɑnsl̩`teʃən] *n.*
　初步診療

4 register [`rɛdʒɪstə] *v.* 登記
5 front desk [`frʌnt`dɛsk] *n.* 櫃檯

Part **2**

第一時間的處理
——急救

10 割傷和擦傷：描述受傷經過

☐ I accidentally¹ cut myself while I was chopping up vegetables.
我切菜時不小心割傷了自己。

☐ I fell off my bike and skinned² my knee.
我從腳踏車摔下來，膝蓋擦破了皮。

☐ I just scraped³ my elbow while rollerblading.⁴ It's not serious.
我溜直排輪時擦傷了手肘。不是很嚴重。

☐ I broke a glass and sliced my finger picking up a broken piece.
我打破了一個玻璃杯，揀碎片時割傷了手指。

☐ This gash⁵ on my forehead won't stop bleeding.
我額頭的傷口不停地流血。

☐ Ouch! I got a paper cut.
唉喲！我被紙割傷了。

Word List ►►►

1 accidentally [ˌæksəˈdɛntḷɪ] *adv.* 偶然地；
  意外地
2 skin [skɪn] *v.* 擦破皮

3 scrape [skrep] *v.* 擦傷
4 rollerblade [ˈrolɚˌbled] *v.* 溜直排輪
5 gash [gæʃ] *n.* 深長的切口（或傷口）

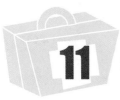

11 割傷和擦傷：治療

☐ **It looks pretty bad. You might need stitches.[1]**
傷口看起來很糟。你可能需要縫幾針。

☐ **There are Band-Aids[2] in the medicine cabinet.**
醫藥箱裡面有 OK 繃。

☐ **You should put some antiseptic cream[3]/ Neosporin on the cut before you use a plaster.[4]**
貼上藥膏之前你應該先在傷口上抹些消毒藥膏／尼奧斯普林。

☐ **Wash the wound with soap and water so it doesn't get infected.[5]**
先將傷口用肥皂和水清洗乾淨，這樣才不會感染。

☐ **If you use a waterproof bandage,[6] it'll heal faster.**
如果你使用防水繃帶，傷口會好得比較快。

☐ **Don't pick at your scab![7]**
不要剝你的結痂！

Word List ▶ ▶ ▶

1 stitches [ˋstɪtʃɪz] *n.* （傷口）縫針
2 Band-Aid [ˋbænd͵ed] *n.* OK 繃
3 antiseptic [͵æntəˋsɛptɪk] cream *n.* 抗菌藥膏
4 plaster [ˋplæstɚ] *n.* 貼布

5 infected [ɪnˋfɛktɪd] *adj.* （傷口）受感染的
6 bandage [ˋbændɪdʒ] *n.* 繃帶
7 scab [skæb] *n.* 痂

第一時間的處理

12 瘀傷：描述受傷經過

☐ I banged[1] my knee on the coffee table.
我的膝蓋撞到了咖啡桌。

☐ I stubbed[2] my toe.
我踢傷了腳趾頭。

☐ I got a bump on my forehead when I fell out of my bed this morning, but it's turned into a bruise.[3]
今天早上我從床上摔下來額頭撞了個包，結果卻變成瘀青。

☐ I bruised my arm so badly that the bruise now has blood spots.
我手臂上的瘀傷非常嚴重，現在都變成血斑了。

☐ Is it normal for a bruise to turn green?
瘀青變成綠色是正常的嗎？

☐ He gave me a black eye![4]
他打得我眼睛瘀青！

Word List ▶▶▶

1 bang [bæŋ] *v.* 猛擊；撞傷
2 stub [stʌb] *v.* 使碰踢

3 bruise [bruz] *n.* 瘀傷；青腫
4 black eye [`blæk`aɪ] *n.* 黑眼圈

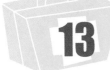

13 瘀傷：治療

☐ Put some ice on it to stop the bruise from getting bigger.
瘀傷處用冰敷以防止擴散。

☐ You should use an ice pack[1] or a cold compress.[2]
你應該使用冰枕或冷敷布。

☐ It will fade[3] on its own. Just give it a few weeks.
瘀青會自行消散。給它幾個禮拜的時間。

☐ You can use a heat pack[4] after two days to make it heal faster.
兩天後你可以用熱敷包讓瘀青快一點消散。

☐ I've heard that if you bruise your leg, you should elevate[5] it during the first day.
我聽人說如果你的腳瘀傷了，在第一天的時候應該把腳抬高。

☐ They say slap a raw steak[6] on your eye to make the swelling[7] go down.
聽說在眼睛貼上生肉片可以消腫。

Word List ▶▶▶

1 ice pack [`aɪs͵pæk] *n.* 冰枕

2 cold compress [kold `kɑmprɛs] *n.* （消炎等用的）冷敷布

3 fade [fed] *v.* 褪去

4 heat pack [`hit͵pæk] *n.* 熱敷包

5 elevate [`ɛlə͵vet] *v.* 舉起；抬起

6 steak [stek] *n.* 厚肉片（尤指牛排）

7 swelling [`swɛlɪŋ] *n.* 腫脹

14 流鼻血：描述經過

☐ Can you please hand me a tissue? My nose is bleeding.
可不可以請你遞張衛生紙給我？我流鼻血了。

☐ I get nosebleeds[1] whenever the air is too dry.
每當空氣太乾燥的時候我就會流鼻血。

☐ This always happens when I'm really stressed.
每次只要我壓力大就會這樣。

☐ I get chronic[2] nosebleeds in the winter.
在冬天我會習慣性流鼻血。

☐ I've been blowing my nose too hard. Now I've got a nosebleed.
我一直擤鼻子擤得太用力了。這會兒流鼻血了。

☐ It's been ten minutes but the bleeding still hasn't stopped.
已經十分鐘了，但血還是流個不停。

Word List ▶ ▶ ▶

1 nosebleed [`noz͵blid] *n.* 流鼻血

2 chronic [`krɑnɪk] *adj.*（病）慢性的；（人）久病的

15 流鼻血：治療

☐ Tilt[1] your head back.
把你的頭向後傾。

☐ Bring your head down and pinch[2] your nostrils[3] together.
低頭，然後捏住鼻孔。

☐ Use a tissue and hold the bridge[4] of your nose.
用張衛生紙按住你的鼻樑。

☐ Ice will help stop the blood flow.
冰塊有助於止血。

☐ You should get a humidifier[5] for your room.
你的房間應該擺一部增濕機。

☐ If it doesn't stop bleeding in the next ten minutes, you should go see a doctor.
如果過了十分鐘血還是流個不停，你就應該去看醫生。

2 第一時間的處理

Word List ▶▶▶

1 tilt [tɪlt] v. 傾斜；偏斜
2 pinch [pɪntʃ] v. 捏；擰
3 nostrils [`nɑstrɪlz] n. 鼻孔
4 bridge [brɪdʒ] n. 鼻樑
5 humidifier [hju`mɪdə,faɪə] n. 濕潤器；增濕器

16 燒燙傷：描述受傷經過

☐ I burned my wrist[1] when I was ironing.
我熨衣服的時候燙傷了手腕。

☐ I scalded[2] myself with hot water.
我被熱水燙傷了。

☐ Michael accidentally jabbed[3] me with a lit cigarette.
麥可不小心用點燃的香菸戳到我。

☐ I singed[4] my hair lighting candles.
我點蠟燭的時候燒到了頭髮。

☐ He spilled[5] a cup of hot coffee on my lap.[6]
他把一杯熱咖啡灑到我的大腿上。

☐ I think I got a really bad burn. It's starting to blister.[7]
我想我的燙傷很嚴重。已經開始起水泡了。

Word List ▶▶▶

1 wrist [rɪst] *n.* 腕；腕關節
2 scald [skɔld] *v.* 燙傷
3 jab [dʒæb] *v.* 刺；戳
4 singe [sɪndʒ] *v.* 把……微微燒焦

5 spill [spɪl] *v.* 濺出；溢出
6 lap [læp] *n.* （腰以下到膝為止的）大腿部
7 blister [ˋblɪstə] *v.* 起水泡

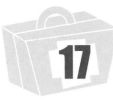

17 燒燙傷：治療

☐ Hold your hand under cold water for a few minutes.
把你的手浸泡在冷水裡面幾分鐘。

☐ Don't put ice on it. It might make it worse.
不要冰敷。那樣可能會讓傷口更嚴重。

☐ We should wrap up your hand with gauze.[1]
我們應該用紗布把你的手包紮起來。

☐ If it really hurts, you can take a pain reliever.[2]
如果傷口真的很痛，你可以吃顆止痛藥。

☐ Don't break the blisters.[3] You could get an infection.[4]
不要弄破水泡，你可能會受到感染。

☐ Make sure you change the gauze every day.
紗布一定要每天更換。

Word List ▶▶▶

1 gauze [gɔz] *n.* （醫用）紗布
2 pain reliever [`pen rɪ`livə] *n.* 止痛藥
3 blister [`blɪstə] *n.* （皮膚上因燙傷、摩擦而起的）水泡

4 infection [ɪn`fɛkʃən] *n.* 傳染；感染

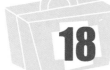

18 曬傷：描述經過

☐ I forgot to use sun block[1] and now I'm as red as a lobster.
我忘了使用防曬乳液，結果現在人紅得像隻龍蝦。

☐ My skin is bubbling.[2] Is that bad?
我的皮膚起水泡了。這樣是不是很糟？

☐ My shoulders got roasted.[3]
我的肩膀曬傷了。

☐ My skin itches[4] and I think my face is all puffy.[5]
我的皮膚很癢，我覺得我的臉整個腫起來了。

☐ I feel really faint.[6] I think I've been out in the sun for too long.
我覺得頭好暈。我想我在太陽底下待太久了。

☐ My arms got sunburned a few days ago, and now the skin is peeling.[7]
我的手臂幾天前曬傷了，現在開始脫皮了。

Word List ▶ ▶ ▶

1 sun block [ˈsʌn͵blɑk] *n.* 防曬乳
2 bubble [ˈbʌbl̩] *v.* 起（水）泡
3 roast [rost] *v.* 烤；炙
4 itch [ɪtʃ] *v.* 發癢

5 puffy [ˈpʌfɪ] *adj.* 脹大的
6 faint [fent] *adj.* 頭暈的
7 peel [pil] *v.* 脫皮

MP3 ▸▸ 019

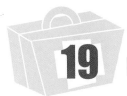

19 曬傷：治療

□ Use aloe vera[1] to help soothe[2] your skin.
用蘆薈露舒緩你的肌膚。

□ Keep slathering[3] on moisturizer[4] to prevent your skin from peeling.
在皮膚上不斷塗抹保濕霜以防止脫皮。

□ Get out of the sun and cover up!
不要站在太陽下，把自己遮蓋起來！

□ Try applying cold compresses soaked in milk and water.
試試牛奶跟水裡浸泡過的冷敷布。

□ You might feel more comfortable if you take a cool bath.
洗個冷水澡你或許會覺得舒服一些。

□ You look like you have sun poisoning.[5] You should stay out of the sun for a few days.
你看起來像是曬傷了。你應該幾天不要再曬太陽。

Word List ▸▸▸

1 aloe vera [ˋælo ˋvɛrə] *n.* 蘆薈（露）
2 soothe [suð] *v.* 緩和
3 slather [ˋslæðɚ] *v.* 厚厚塗一層；大量塗抹
4 moisturizer [ˋmɔɪstʃə͵raɪzɚ] *n.* 保濕霜
5 sun poisoning [ˋsʌn͵pɔɪzn̩ɪŋ] *n.* 皮膚因紫外線照射而受傷

20 起疹子：描述經過

☐ I think I got a rash[1] from eating those shrimp.
我想我因為吃了那些蝦子而起了疹子。

☐ I can't stop scratching[2] my arm. This rash itches like crazy.
我忍不住一直搔手臂。這疹子癢得要命。

☐ I think my rash is spreading.[3]
我想我的疹子在擴散。

☐ I've never had a rash like this before. I usually get small red bumps, but this is one huge welt.[4]
我以前疹子從沒起得這麼嚴重。我通常只是冒些小紅點，但現在卻腫成這麼一大條。

☐ I think I might have sat in poison ivy.[5]
我想我可能坐到野葛了。

☐ Cats make me break out[6] in hives.[7]
貓會讓我起蕁麻疹。

Word List ▶▶▶

1 rash [ræʃ] n. 疹子
2 scratch [skrætʃ] v. 抓；搔
3 spread [sprɛd] v. 蔓延；散佈
4 welt [wɛlt] n. 條狀紅腫
5 poison ivy [ˋpɔɪzn̩ ˋaɪvɪ] n. 野葛；櫟葉毒漆樹
6 break out 爆發；突然發生
7 hives [haɪvz] n. 蕁麻疹

21 起疹子：治療

☐ For irritation[1] caused by poison ivy you can use calamine[2] lotion.
因野葛產生的不適可以塗爐甘石藥膏。

☐ Scratching spreads rashes.
抓會使得疹子擴散。

☐ Try using some ice to make it stop itching.
試試用冰敷止癢。

☐ Rashes are sometimes caused by toxins[3] in your body, so drink plenty of water to flush them out.
疹子有時候是你體內的毒素所引起的，所以喝大量的水可以把它們排掉。

☐ That looks like a heat rash. Wear loose, comfortable clothing.
這看起來像汗疹。穿寬鬆、舒適的衣服。

☐ Don't take really hot showers.
不要洗太熱的澡。

Word List ▶▶▶

1 irritation [ˌɪrəˋteʃən] n. 發炎；斑疹；疼痛
2 calamine [ˋkæləˌmaɪn] n. （藥用）爐甘石
3 toxin [ˋtɑksɪn] n. 毒素

22 蚊蟲或動物叮咬：描述經過

☐ I'm getting eaten by mosquitoes out here!
我快要被這裡的蚊子咬死了！

☐ These don't look like mosquito bites. What do you think bit me?
這些看起來不像是被蚊子叮的。你覺得我被什麼叮了？

☐ I got stung by a bee / wasp.[1]
我被蜜蜂／黃蜂螫到了。

☐ I think I'm having an allergic[2] reaction to this insect bite.
我想我對這種昆蟲叮咬起了過敏反應。

☐ That cat / dog just bit me on the ankle![3]
那隻貓／狗剛剛咬了我的腳踝！

☐ I was walking in the woods and something bit me!
我剛剛在林間散步時被什麼東西給咬了！

Word List ▸▸▸

1 wasp [wɑsp] *n.* 黃蜂
2 allergic [ɚˋlɝdʒɪk] *adj.* 過敏的

3 ankle [ˋæŋkl̩] *n.* 踝；足踝

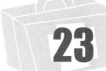

23 蚊蟲或動物叮咬：治療

☐ You should use some insect repellent[1] whenever you're outdoors for a long time.

只要長時間待在戶外就應該使用驅蟲劑。

☐ You could have been bitten by a flea[2] or a tick.[3]

你可能是被跳蚤或壁蝨叮咬了。

☐ Make sure you get the stinger[4] out.

務必把螫針拔除。

☐ You can try putting an antihistamine[5] on the bite.

你可以在被叮咬處塗上抗組織胺藥試試。

☐ When was the last time you got a tetanus[6] shot?

你上一次打破傷風針是什麼時候？

☐ You should see a doctor immediately, because animals like raccoons[7] and bats often have rabies.[8]

你應該立刻去看醫生，因為浣熊或蝙蝠之類的動物常常有狂犬病。

Word List ▶▶▶

1 insect repellent [ˋɪnsɛkt rɪˏpɛlənt] *n.* 驅蟲劑
2 flea [fli] *n.* 跳蚤
3 tick [tɪk] *n.* 壁蝨
4 stinger [ˋstɪŋɚ] *n.* 螫針

5 antihistamine [ˏæntɪˋhɪstəmin] *n.* 抗組胺劑
6 tetanus [ˋtɛtənəs] *n.* 破傷風
7 raccoon [ræˋkun] *n.* 浣熊
8 rabies [ˋrebiz] *n.* 狂犬病

24 感染：描述經過

☐ I think my cut got infected.
我想我的傷口感染了。

☐ My wound is leaking yellow fluid.[1] Is that bad?
我的傷口有黃色液體流出。這樣嚴不嚴重？

☐ I have a sore throat[2] that just won't go away.
我喉嚨痛，一直好不了。

☐ I think I got an ear infection from swimming in the river.
我想我在河裡游泳的時候耳朵受到了感染。

☐ I have a sore[3] on my back that keeps getting bigger.
我的背上長了腫瘡，愈變愈大。

☐ My eye is really red and swollen.[4]
我的眼睛真的很紅又腫。

Word List ▶▶▶

1 fluid [`fluɪd] *n.* 流質；液體
2 sore throat [`sor `θrot] *n.* 喉嚨痛
3 sore [sor] *n.* 腫瘡
4 swollen [`swolən] *adj.* 膨脹的；浮腫的

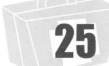

25 感染：治療

☐ Wash it out and then apply an antibiotic[1] cream.
將傷口清洗乾淨，然後塗上抗生素藥膏。

☐ Yeah, if there's yellow or green pus,[2] then it's infected.
沒錯，如果流出黃色或綠色的膿，就表示傷口被感染了。

☐ You might have tonsillitis.[3] You should see a doctor.
你可能得了扁桃腺炎。你應該去看醫生。

☐ I'll take you to the pharmacy[4] to get you some ear drops.[5]
我帶你去藥局買瓶耳藥水。

☐ You might have a staph[6] infection. If it gets worse, you'll have to take antibiotics.
你可能被葡萄球菌感染。如果惡化，你就必須服用抗生素。

☐ I think you have pinkeye.[7] The doctor can tell you how to treat it.
我想你得了急性結膜炎。醫生會告訴你該怎麼處理。

Word List ▶▶▶

1 antibiotic [ˌæntɪbaɪˋɑtɪk] n. 抗生素
2 pus [pʌs] n. 膿
3 tonsillitis [ˌtɑnsḷˋaɪtɪs] n. 扁桃腺炎
4 pharmacy [ˋfɑrməsɪ] n. 藥房
5 ear drops [ˋɪrˌdrɑps] n. 耳藥水
6 staph [stæf] n. 葡萄球菌
　（= staphylococcus [ˌstæfələˋkɑkəs]）
7 pinkeye [ˋpɪŋkˌaɪ] n. 急性結膜炎

26 扭傷或拉傷：描述經過

☐ I missed the last step and twisted[1] my ankle.
我沒踏到最後一個階梯，結果扭傷了腳踝。

☐ I heard a popping[2] sound when I fell down.
我跌倒的時候聽到啪的一聲。

☐ I can't bend my elbow.
我的手肘不能彎。

☐ It really hurts when I walk.
我走路的時候真的很痛。

☐ I think I slept funny. My neck really hurts.
我想我睡覺姿勢不良。我的脖子真的好痛。

☐ I pulled a muscle[3] playing basketball last night.
我昨晚打籃球的時候肌肉拉傷了。

Word List ▶ ▶ ▶

1 twist [twɪst] *v.* 扭傷
2 popping [ˋpɑpɪŋ] *adj.* 發出啪聲的

3 muscle [ˋmʌsl̩] *n.* 肌肉

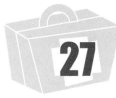

27 扭傷或拉傷：治療

☐ Try not to put any weight[1] on it for the next day or two.
未來這一、兩天儘量不要讓患部承受重力。

☐ Ice it to make the swelling go down.
冰敷患部以消腫。

☐ It doesn't look like it's broken, but you should still see a doctor.
看起來骨頭沒有斷，但是你還是應該去看醫生。

☐ You can use an ankle brace[2] to give you extra support.
你可以穿護踝加強支撐。

☐ Elevating your leg will help bring down the swelling.
把腳抬高有助於消腫。

☐ I usually massage a pulled muscle with ice for about twenty minutes.
我通常會用冰塊按摩拉傷的肌肉大約二十分鐘。

Word List ▶▶▶

1 weight [wet] *n.* 重量

2 ankle brace [ˋæŋkl̩ˏbres] *n.* 護踝

2
第一時間的處理

Part 3

非處方治療——
購買成藥

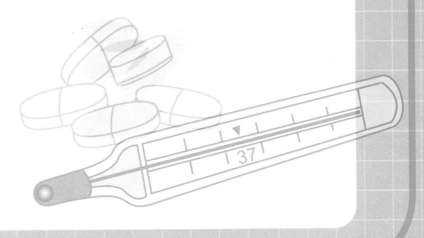

28 上哪兒找藥品——詢問

在許多西方國家，人們如果只是著涼或得了流行性感冒，通常不會看醫生。他們會購買在多數藥妝店或藥局都買得到的非處方用藥。以下教你該怎麼說出自己的需求。

☐ Hi, I'm looking for eyedrops.[1]
你好，我在找眼藥水。

☐ Excuse me, where can I find the Band-Aids?
對不起，請問 *OK* 繃放在哪裡？

☐ Do you know where the cough drops[2] are?
你知不知道止咳錠在哪裡？

☐ Could you point me in the direction of the vitamins?
你可不可以指一下放維他命的地方？

☐ (*pointing to a list*) Could you please help me find this?
（指著一張單子）可否請你幫我找這個東西？

☐ Which aisle[3] can I find aspirin[4] in?
阿斯匹靈在哪一排走道？

Word List ▶ ▶ ▶

1 eyedrops [ˈaɪˌdrɑps] *n.* 眼藥水
2 cough drop [ˈkɔf ˌdrɑp] *n.* 止咳錠；喉糖
3 aisle [aɪl] *n.* 走道
4 aspirin [ˈæspərɪn] *n.* 阿斯匹靈（藥片）

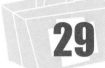

29 上哪兒找藥品——回答

☐ It's at the end of aisle 3.
在第三排走道盡頭。

☐ Take the first aisle and it'll be on your right.[1]
走第一排走道，東西就放在你的右手邊。

☐ Go all the way to the back and you'll find it in the corner.[2]
一直走到後面，東西就放在角落上。

☐ It should be with all the other pain relievers.
它應該和所有其他的止痛藥放在一起。

☐ I actually don't know. Let me ask someone for you.
其實我不太清楚。我幫你問其他人。

☐ Follow me. I'll show you where it is.
跟我來。我告訴你放在什麼地方。

3
非
處
方
治
療

Word List ▶▶▶

1 on your right 在你的右邊

2 corner [ˋkɔrnɚ] n. 角落

30 尋求適當的醫療方式——詢問

☐ Do you have anything for a really bad cough?[1]
你們有沒有什麼藥可以治療嚴重的咳嗽？

☐ I might have a fever.[2] Is there anything that can make it go down?
我好像發燒了。有什麼藥可以退燒嗎？

☐ What can you recommend for cold sores?[3]
你會建議用什麼藥治療唇皰疹？

☐ Is there something I can take for a really stuffy nose?[4]
我嚴重鼻塞，有沒有什麼藥可以吃？

☐ I can't sleep at night because I get coughing fits.[5]
我晚上睡不著，因為我一直咳嗽。

☐ What can I take for an upset[6] stomach?
我胃不舒服，可以吃什麼藥？

Word List ▶ ▶ ▶

1 bad cough　嚴重咳嗽

2 fever [`fivɚ] n. 發燒

3 cold sore [`kold ˌsor] n. 唇皰疹

4 stuffy nose [`stʌfɪ `noz] n. 鼻塞

5 fit [fɪt] n.（病的）發作

6 upset [ʌp`sɛt] adj. 不舒服的

31 建議適當的醫療方式——回答

☐ Here, this nighttime formula[1] will help you get a good night's rest.
諾，這個安眠藥劑會讓你一夜好眠。

☐ This cough medicine is a pain reliever and cough suppressant.[2]
這個咳嗽藥方是止痛藥兼鎮咳劑。

☐ If you just have a mild[3] fever, a few Advil[4] or Tylenol[5] tablets will help.
如果你只是輕微發燒，吃一點 Advil 或 Tylenol 藥片會有幫助。

☐ We have a few different sinus[6] medicines. Do you have a stuffy nose because of a cold or allergies?[7]
我們有幾種不同鼻竇藥。你的鼻塞是因為感冒還是過敏所引起的？

☐ If you're feeling nauseous,[8] you should take Pepto Bismol,[9] but an antacid[10] will work for a regular upset stomach.
如果你覺得噁心，可以吃 Pepto Bismol，但是一般的胃不舒服用制酸劑就可以了。

☐ We have a gel[11] and an ointment[12] that helps cold sores.
我們有凝膠和軟膏可以治療唇皰疹。

Word List ▶▶▶

1 formula [ˋfɔrmjələ] n. 配方；處方
2 suppressant [səˋprɛsn̩t] n. 抑制藥
3 mild [maɪld] adj. 輕微的
4 Advil [ˋædvɪl] n. 感冒與止痛藥
5 Tylenol [ˋtaɪlənɔl] n.【商標】泰熱諾（感冒與止痛藥）
6 sinus [ˋsaɪnəs] n. 鼻竇
7 allergy [ˋælədʒɪ] n. 過敏症
8 nauseous [ˋnɔʃɪəs] adj. 令人作嘔的；使人厭惡的
9 Pepto Bismol [ˋpɛptoˋbɪzmol] n. 胃藥
10 antacid [æntˋæsɪd] n. 解酸劑；抗酸劑
11 gel [dʒɛl] n. 凝膠
12 ointment [ˋɔɪntmənt] n. 軟膏；藥膏

32 用藥諮詢──詢問

☐ Will this medicine make me feel sleepy?
這個藥會讓人昏昏欲睡嗎？

☐ How many capsules¹ do I take each day?
我一天要服用幾顆膠囊？

☐ How much medicine do I take each time?
我藥每次要吃多少？

☐ Is it better to take this before or after a meal?
這種藥飯前還是飯後吃比較好？

☐ Is it safe to apply² this gel on my lip?
這種凝膠塗在嘴唇上安全嗎？

☐ How long can I use this for?
這種藥我可以用多久？

Word List ▶▶▶

1 capsule [`kæps!] *n.* 膠囊

2 apply [ə`plaɪ] *v.* 塗；敷

33 用藥諮詢──回答

☐ Take two capsules, three times a day.

每次吃兩顆膠囊，一天三次。

☐ Just use the ointment until the rash goes down.

就塗藥膏，直到疹子消失為止。

☐ Take the medicine after each meal, and once before you go to bed.

藥每餐飯後吃，睡前再吃一次。

☐ This medicine is safe to ingest.[1]

這種藥吃下去很安全。

☐ If it doesn't clear up[2] in a few days, you should probably see a doctor.

如果幾天之內沒有痊癒，你或許就該去看醫生。

☐ It's a non-drowsy[3] formula, so you should be able to take it during the day.

這是不嗜睡的處方，所以你應該可以白天吃。

Word List ▶▶▶

1 ingest [ɪnˋdʒɛst] v. 攝取；吸收
2 clear up 減輕；痊癒
3 drowsy [ˋdraʊzɪ] adj. 昏昏欲睡的

Part **4**

醫院／診所管理

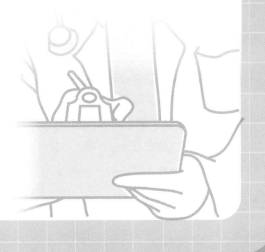

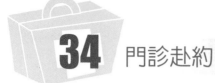

34 門診赴約

你可以這樣說

- Hi, I'm here to see Dr. Warner.
  嗨，我來看華納醫生的門診。

- I have a 2 o'clock appointment with Dr. Newton.
  我和牛頓醫師預約兩點的門診。

- Excuse me. I've been waiting for my appointment for forty-five minutes already. When will I be able to see the doctor?
  對不起。我等我預約的門診已經四十五分鐘了。我什麼時候才可以看得到醫生？

對方可能這樣回答

- Please take a seat.[1] She'll be right with you.
  請坐，她很快就來。

- Go right in. The doctor's expecting[2] you.
  請直接進去，醫師正在等你。

- I'm sorry. We're a little backed up.[3] It shouldn't be too much longer.
  對不起，人稍微多了些。應該不會再等太久了。

Word List ▶▶▶

1 Please take a seat. 請坐。　　　　　3 back up 人或車輛在隊伍中越積越多
2 expect [ɪk`spɛkt] v. 期待；盼望

35 臨時就診

你可以這樣問

☐ I'd like to see the GP[1] on duty[2] today.
我想看今天有看診的普通科醫師。

☐ How long do you think I'll have to wait?
你看我必須等多久？

☐ What time do you see patients[3] until?
這裡看診最晚到什麼時候？

對方可能這樣回答

☐ Certainly. Please take a number and fill out[4] these forms.[5]
好的。請取號碼牌，並填妥這些表格。

☐ There are eight people ahead of[6] you, so I'd say at least an hour.
你前面還有八個人，所以我想至少還需要一小時。

☐ Please take a seat until your number is called.
請坐，等到你的號碼被叫到。

Word List ▶ ▶ ▶

1 GP = general practitioner 全科（普通）醫生（與專科醫師相對）
2 on duty 值班；上班
3 patient [`peʃənt] n. 病人
4 fill out 填寫
5 form [fɔrm] n. 表格
6 ahead of 在……之前

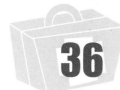

ABC Hospital Admission Form

Date: .... / .... / ....
(year) (month) (day)

Last Name: ....

First Name: .... M.I.:[1] ....

Mailing Address:[2] ....

City: .... State:................ Zipcode: ....

Home Address (if different from above)

....

City: .... State: .... Zipcode: ....

Home Phone Number: ....

Birthdate: ....(year)/...............(month)/...............(day)

Social Security Number:[3] ....

Sex: .... Martial Status:[4] ....

ABC 醫院就診表

日期：......... / .... / ....
(年)　　(月)　　(日)

名字：...

姓氏：... 中間名的起首字母：.........................

通訊地址：...

城市：.......................... 州別：.................. 郵遞區號：..................

住家地址（與通訊地址不同者）

....

城市：.......................... 州別：.................. 郵遞區號：..................

住家電話：...

出生日期：....................(年)/...................(月)/...................(日)

社會福利證號碼：...

性別：.............................. 婚姻狀況：...........................

If under 18, please provide parent information. If married, please provide spouse[5] information.

Name: ....

Social Security Number: ....

Employer's Name and Address: ....

....

Have you been treated at this hospital before?　　Yes　　No

Allergies:　　Yes　　No　　Maybe

Allergy Type: Medication　　Food　　Latex[6]　　Others: ....

Emergency Contact: ....

Relationship to Patient:[7] ....

Address: ....

City: ....　State:...............　Zipcode: ....

Daytime Phone: ....　Evening Phone: ....

Please list any other special needs or physical limitations[8] the hospital staff should know about.

如果未滿十八歲，請填寫父母姓名。如果已婚，請填寫配偶姓名。

姓名：..

社會福利證號碼：..

雇主姓名和電話：..

....

以前是否曾在本院就診？　　有　　沒有

過敏：　　有　　　沒有　　可能有

過敏類型：　　藥物　　食物　　乳膠　　其他：..........................

緊急聯絡人：..

與病人的關係：..

地址：..

城市：.......................... 州別：.............. 郵遞區號：..............

白天聯絡電話：........................ 晚上聯絡電話：....................

請列出其他任何醫務人員應該知道的特殊需求或身體狀況。

....

37 填寫表格——關鍵字彙和建議

訣竅

√ 用正楷書寫清楚。

√ 選擇萬一發生狀況時,你希望可以立即通知的緊急聯絡人。

√ 務必寫下是否對任何藥物過敏,並提供醫護人員任何詳細記載你過敏情
形的文件(病歷表、信件、紀錄等)。

關鍵字彙

1 M.I. (middle initial) 中間名字的起首字母

2 Mailing Address 通訊地址
如果醫院要寄信給你,會用到這個地址。

3 Social Security Number 社會福利證號碼
常用 SS# 表示。這相當於美國人的身分證號碼。記得寫下你的護照號
碼,並且詢問醫護人員是否還有其他院方可能需要知道的資訊。

4 Martial Status 婚姻狀況

5 spouse [spaʊz] n. 配偶

6 latex [ˋletɛks] n. (橡膠樹等的)乳汁

7 Relationship to Patient 與病人的關係
指你和緊急聯絡人之間的關係。緊急聯絡人通常是配偶(先生/妻子)、
父親或母親、好友。

8 Special Needs / Physical Limitations 特殊需求/身體狀況
醫院必須知道你是否需要特殊協助或者行動是否自如。例如:他們必須
知道你是否坐輪椅,或是否罹患了會影響日常作息的疾病。

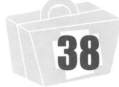

38 保險事宜——詢問

☐ Do I need to ask my insurance company[1] before I can make an appointment?

我預約之前是否需要先詢問我的保險公司？

☐ I have travel insurance.[2] Will it cover[3] my expenses?[4]

我有投保旅遊險。能不能涵蓋我的費用？

☐ Do I need insurance to see a doctor here?

在這裡我必須有保險才能看醫生嗎？

☐ Will you bill[5] my insurance company directly?

你們會將帳單直接開給我的保險公司嗎？

☐ How much will this cost if my insurance won't cover it?

萬一我的保險不支付這個費用，那我要付多少錢？

☐ I only have my country's national health insurance.[6]

我只保了自己國家的全民健康保險。

Word List ▶▶▶

1 insurance company [ɪnˋʃʊrənsˋkʌmpənɪ]
   n. 保險公司
2 travel insurance 旅遊保險
3 cover [ˋkʌvə] v. （保險範圍）涵蓋；（保險）
   支付

4 expense [ɪkˋspɛns] n. 費用；價錢
5 bill [bɪl] v. 將……記爲（某人）的帳；給……
   …開帳單
6 National Health Insurance 全民健康保險

39 保險事宜——回答

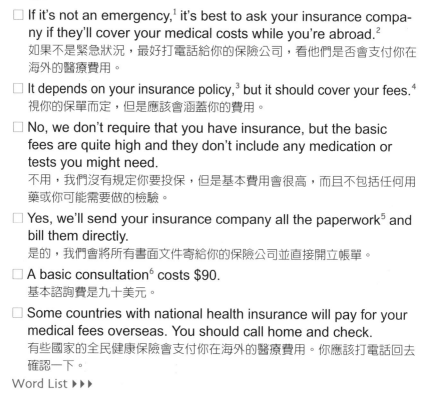

☐ If it's not an emergency,[1] it's best to ask your insurance company if they'll cover your medical costs while you're abroad.[2]
如果不是緊急狀況，最好打電話給你的保險公司，看他們是否會支付你在海外的醫療費用。

☐ It depends on your insurance policy,[3] but it should cover your fees.[4]
視你的保單而定，但是應該會涵蓋你的費用。

☐ No, we don't require that you have insurance, but the basic fees are quite high and they don't include any medication or tests you might need.
不用，我們沒有規定你要投保，但是基本費用會很高，而且不包括任何用藥或你可能需要做的檢驗。

☐ Yes, we'll send your insurance company all the paperwork[5] and bill them directly.
是的，我們會將所有書面文件寄給你的保險公司並直接開立帳單。

☐ A basic consultation[6] costs $90.
基本諮詢費是九十美元。

☐ Some countries with national health insurance will pay for your medical fees overseas. You should call home and check.
有些國家的全民健康保險會支付你在海外的醫療費用。你應該打電話回去確認一下。

Word List ▶▶▶

1 emergency [ɪˋmɝdʒənsɪ] n. 緊急情況
2 abroad [əˋbrɔd] adv. 在國外
3 policy [ˋpɑləsɪ] n. 保單
4 fee [fi] n. 費用
5 paperwork [ˋpepɚ͵wɝk] n. 文書工作；書面文件
6 consultation [͵kɑnsḷˋteʃən] n. 諮詢

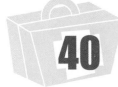

40 付款——詢問

☐ Will you bill my insurance company or me first?

你們會將帳單先寄給我的保險公司還是先寄給我？

☐ Do you accept[1] credit cards?[2]

你們接不接受信用卡付款？

☐ Would it be okay if I wrote you a check?[3]

我開支票給你們可以嗎？

☐ (*looking at the receipt[4]*) What's this fee for?

（看著收據）這個費用是做什麼的？

☐ I'll just pay with cash.[5]

我付現好了。

☐ Does this bill cover everything?

這帳單包含所有項目嗎？

Word List ▶▶▶

1 accept [əkˋsɛpt] *v.* 接受

2 credit card 信用卡

3 check [tʃɛk] *n.* 支票

4 receipt [rɪˋsit] *n.* 收據

5 cash [kæʃ] *n.* 現金

41 付款——回答

☐ You'll receive a separate[1] bill from your physician.[2]

你的醫師會另外寄一張帳單給你。

☐ Yes, we accept all major credit cards.

是的，我們接受所有主要的信用卡。

☐ A personal check is fine, but you'll need to show identification.[3]

個人支票可以，但是你必須出示身分證件。

☐ There's an ATM[4] located in the lobby[5] if you need it.

如果你需要的話，大廳那裡有台自動提款機。

☐ It's the fee for your test.

這是你的檢驗費用。

☐ We'll verify[6] with your insurance company about payment[7] first.

我們會先和你的保險公司確認付款事宜。

Word List ▶ ▶ ▶

1 separate [ˋsɛpəˏrɪt] *adj.* 分開的

2 physician [fɪˋzɪʃən] *n.* 內科醫生；醫師

3 identification [aɪˏdɛntəfəˋkeʃən] *n.* 身分證明

4 ATM = Automated Teller Machine 自動存提款機

5 lobby [ˋlɑbɪ] *n.* 大廳

6 verify [ˋvɛrəˏfaɪ] *v.* 證實；確認

7 payment [ˋpemənt] *n.* 支付（的款項）

Part 5

診療第一步——
和醫師對談

42 醫師的問候語

你的醫生可能會提出一些問題以便正確診斷你的疾病。儘可能提供醫護人員充分的訊息，不用害怕提出你的疑問。如果覺得你的醫生不太關心，不要遲疑，去請教其他健康照護專業人員。

☐ Hi. I'm Dr. Kim. How are you feeling today?
嗨，我是金姆醫師。你今天覺得如何？

☐ What seems to be the problem?
大概是什麼問題？

☐ Where does it hurt?
哪裡痛？

☐ What are your symptoms?[1]
你有什麼症狀？

☐ Are you taking any medication?
你是不是有在服用任何藥物？

☐ How long have you been having this problem?
你這個毛病有多久了？

Word List ▶▶▶

1 symptom [`sɪmptəm] *n.* 徵狀；病的症狀

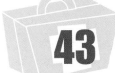

43 解釋哪裡不舒服

☐ Not very well, I'm afraid.
恐怕不是太好。

☐ I have a high fever.
我發高燒。

☐ I have a pain in my shoulders and back.
我肩膀和背都痛。

☐ I've been feeling nauseous[1] since this morning.
我從今天早上開始就一直想吐。

☐ I just took some aspirin.
我剛剛吃了些阿斯匹靈。

☐ I started feeling sick Sunday night.
從星期天晚上開始就覺得不舒服。

Word List ▸▸▸

1 nauseous [`nɔʃɪəs] *adj.* 令人作嘔的；使人厭惡的

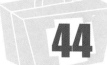

44 感冒／流行性感冒──醫護人員詢問

☐ **Do you have a runny[1] or stuffy nose?**
你是流鼻水還是鼻塞？

☐ **Any aches[2] or pains?**
哪裡疼痛或不舒服？

☐ **Are you experiencing a dry cough?[3]**
你是不是有乾咳？

☐ **Are you coughing up any phlegm?[4]**
你咳嗽有沒有痰？

☐ **Does it hurt to swallow?[5]**
吞嚥的時候會不會痛？

☐ **Are you feeling feverish?[6]**
你是不是覺得有點發燒？

Word List ▸▸▸

1 runny [ˋrʌnɪ] *adj.* 流鼻涕的
2 ache [ek] *n.* 疼痛
3 dry cough [kɔf] *n.* 乾咳

4 phlegm [flɛm] *n.* 痰
5 swallow [ˋswɑlo] *v.* 嚥下；吞下
6 feverish [ˋfivərɪʃ] *adj.* 發燒的

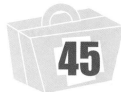

45 感冒／流行性感冒──你可以這樣回答

☐ I started feeling tired three days ago.

我三天前開始覺得疲倦。

☐ I can't stop sneezing.[1]

我一直不停地打噴嚏。

☐ The mucus[2] in my nose has turned from yellow to green.

我鼻子裡的黏液從黃色變成了綠色。

☐ I'm coughing up clear phlegm.

我咳出的是清痰。

☐ My sore throat is worse in the morning.

我的喉嚨痛今天早上變得更嚴重了。

☐ I took my temperature and I think I have a mild fever.

我量過體溫了，我想我有一點發燒。

5
診療第一步

Word List ▶▶▶

1 sneeze [sniz] *v.* 打噴嚏　　　　2 mucus [ˋmjukəs] *n.* 黏液

46 頭痛——醫護人員詢問

☐ **When did the headaches first start?**
第一次頭痛是什麼時候開始的？

☐ **Do they last a long time?**
頭痛是不是持續很久？

☐ **Is it a dull[1] ache or a piercing[2] pain?**
是隱隱作痛，還是頭痛欲裂？

☐ **Where is the pain located?**
痛的位置在哪裡？

☐ **When do they usually occur?**
頭痛通常發生在什麼時候？

☐ **Do you have any other symptoms? Vision problems? Tightness in your jaw?[3]**
你還有沒有其他症狀？視覺有沒有問題？下巴有沒有緊緊的？

Word List ▶ ▶ ▶

1 dull [dʌl] v. 隱約的
2 piercing [ˋpɪrsɪŋ] adj. 尖銳的；刺穿的

3 jaw [dʒɔ] n. 下顎

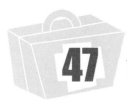

47 頭痛——你可以這樣回答

☐ They started about a week ago.
頭痛大約一個禮拜前開始。

☐ Sometimes it lasts for a few seconds. Other times it lasts for 15 minutes or more.
有時候持續幾秒鐘，有時候持續十五分鐘，甚至更久。

☐ The pain is isolated[1] around my temples.[2]
痛的地方主要在我兩側太陽穴。

☐ It feels like a pounding on the right side of my head.
痛得像我的腦袋右側在乒乒乓乓響。

☐ It's more like a throbbing[3] pain.
感覺比較像是陣陣抽痛。

☐ Whenever I get a headache, my vision[4] gets blurry.[5]
我只要頭痛，視線就會模糊。

5

診療第一步

Word List ▶▶▶

1 isolated [ˋaɪsḷ͵etɪd] *adj.* 被隔離的
2 temple [ˋtɛmpl] *n.* 太陽穴
3 throb [θrɑb] *v.* 心臟、脈搏等的跳動；悸動

4 vision [ˋvɪdʒən] *n.* 視力
5 blurry [ˋblɜɪ] *adj.* 模糊的

48 疼痛不舒服——醫護人員詢問

☐ Is it a muscle[1] pain or a joint[2] pain?
是肌肉疼痛，還是關節痛？

☐ When does it usually hurt?
通常什麼時候會痛？

☐ Does your muscle feel really stiff?[3]
你會覺得肌肉非常僵硬嗎？

☐ Can you move your arm around?
你的手臂可以隨意擺動嗎？

☐ Have you overworked[4] this muscle lately?
你最近這部分肌肉是否運動過度？

☐ If you've already iced[5] it, you can use heat to help soothe[6] the pain.
如果你已經冰敷過了，可以用熱敷來舒緩疼痛。

Word List ▶▶▶

1 muscle [`mʌsl] n. 肌肉
2 joint [dʒɔɪnt] n. 關節
3 stiff [stɪf] adj. 僵硬的
4 overworked [ˌovɚˋwɝkt] adj. 工作過度的
5 ice [aɪs] v. 以冰覆蓋在肌膚上
6 soothe [suð] v. 緩和；減輕

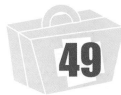

49 疼痛不舒服──你可以這樣回答

☐ It feels like it's coming from my elbow.[1]
疼痛的感覺像是從手肘那邊傳過來的。

☐ It's hard to straighten[2] my leg.
我的腿伸不太直。

☐ My back always hurts after I play golf.
我只要打完高爾夫背就會痛。

☐ I think I threw out[3] my back.
我想我閃到腰了。

☐ I've been resting for three days, but it still really hurts.
我已經休息三天了,但還是很痛。

☐ My muscle feels really tender.[4] Could I have an infection?[5]
我的肌肉一碰就痛。我是不是感染了什麼?

5

診療第一步

Word List ▶ ▶ ▶

1 elbow [ˋɛlbo] *n.* 手肘
2 straighten [ˋstretn̩] *v.* 使變直;拉直
3 throw out one's back 閃到腰

4 tender [ˋtɛndɚ] *adj.* 脆弱的;一觸就痛的
5 infection [ɪnˋfɛkʃən] *n.* 感染

50 消化道問題──醫護人員詢問

☐ **Are you constipated?**[1]

你是不是便秘？

☐ **Do you get heartburn?**[2]

你的胃會不會灼熱？

☐ **Do certain foods make you bloated?**[3]

是不是有某些特定的食物會讓你脹氣？

☐ **You may need to change your diet.**[4]

你可能需要改變你日常的飲食。

☐ **Do you have a lot of gas?**

你肚子裡是不是有很多的氣？

☐ **Is the vomiting associated with**[5] **the gas?**

嘔吐是不是跟排氣有關連？

Word List ▸▸▸

1 constipated [ˋkɑnstəˏpetɪd] *adj.* 患有便秘的
2 heartburn [ˋhɑrtˏbɝn] *n.* 胃灼熱
3 bloated [ˋblotɪd] *adj.* 膨脹的

4 diet [ˋdaɪət] *n.* 日常的飲食
5 associated [əˋsoʃɪˏetɪd] with
　與⋯⋯有關聯的

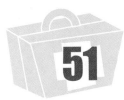
51 消化道問題——你可以這樣回答

☐ I've got a really bad case of diarrhea.[1]
我腹瀉得很嚴重。

☐ I get a pain in my chest when I eat late at night.
我晚上晚一點進食的時候胸口會痛。

☐ I can't seem to stop burping.[2]
我似乎沒法停止打嗝。

☐ I've tried everything to get rid of my bad breath,[3] but nothing
seems to work.
我一直努力想去除口臭，但怎麼做都沒用。

☐ I pass a lot of gas[4] right after a meal.
我吃過飯後會一直放屁。

☐ I can't keep anything down.[5]
我吃什麼就吐什麼。

Word List ▶ ▶ ▶

1 diarrhea [ˌdaɪəˈriə] *n.* 腹瀉
2 burp [bɜp] *v.* 打嗝
3 bad breath 口臭

4 pass gas 放屁
5 keep down （把食物）留在胃中

52 腹部問題——醫護人員詢問

☐ Which side is the pain on?
哪一邊會痛？

☐ If it's on the left, it could be appendicitis.[1]
如果是左邊會痛，可能是盲腸炎。

☐ Does the area feel swollen?
這個部位是否覺得腫脹？

☐ Are you having regular[2] bowel movements?[3]
你的排便正常嗎？

☐ What does your urine[4] look like?
你的尿液是什麼顏色？

☐ Does it hurt to pass stool?[5]
上大號的時候會痛嗎？

Word List ▶▶▶

1 appendicitis [ə͵pɛndə`saɪtɪs] *n.* 闌尾炎；盲腸炎

2 regular [`rɛgjələ] *adj.* 規律的；正常的

3 bowel [`bauəl] *n.* 腸（bowel movement 指排便）

4 urine [`jurɪn] *n.* 尿

5 pass stool [stul] 解便

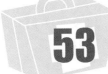

53 腹部問題——你可以這樣回答

☐ **The pain is on my left side.**
痛在我的左側。

☐ **I keep doubling[1] over from the pain.**
我痛到腰挺不起來。

☐ **There's blood in my urine.**
我有血尿。

☐ **It burns when I urinate.[2]**
我小便的時候有灼熱感。

☐ **I get really bad cramps[3] during my period.[4]**
我月經來的時候腹部會嚴重絞痛。

☐ **There's a hard lump[5] on my lower right abdomen.[6]**
我腹部右下方有個硬硬的腫塊。

Word List ▶▶▶

1 double over （因疼痛或笑）而彎著身子
2 urinate [ˋjurəˏnet] v. 排尿
3 cramps [kræmps] n. 腹部絞痛
4 period [ˋpɪrɪəd] n. 經期
5 lump [lʌmp] n. 腫塊；隆起
6 abdomen [ˋæbdəmən] n. 腹部

54 胸部疼痛——醫護人員詢問

☐ Is the pain between your shoulder bones[1] or under your breastbone?[2]

痛是在肩胛骨之間，還是胸骨下方？

☐ What does it feel like?

怎麼個痛法？

☐ Does the pain occur while you're at rest[3] or while you're moving about?

你靜止的時候會痛，還是活動的時候會痛？

☐ Is the pain always in the same place?

是否總是同一個地方在痛？

☐ Does the pain come on[4] suddenly, or does it gradually[5] get stronger?

是突然會很痛，還是慢慢地愈來愈痛？

☐ Does anything you do make the pain worse?

你做什麼事的時候會讓你覺得更痛嗎？

Word List ▶▶▶

1 shoulder bone [`ʃoldə,bon] n. 肩胛骨

2 breastbone [`brɛst,bon] n. 胸骨

3 at rest 靜止

4 come on （病痛的）發作

5 gradually [`grædʒʊəlɪ] adv.
　 逐步地；漸漸地

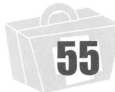
55 胸部疼痛——你可以這樣回答

☐ It's like something is squeezing[1] my heart.
感覺像有東西在擠壓我的心臟。

☐ There's a lot of pressure[2] in the middle of my chest.
胸腔中間壓迫感很重。

☐ The pain moves from my chest to my back.
疼痛從我的前胸傳到我的後背。

☐ It's like something is slowly crushing[3] me.
感覺像有東西在慢慢地輾壓我。

☐ It helps if I rest, but the pain doesn't entirely go away.
如果我休息不動就比較好，但是疼痛並沒有完全消失。

☐ It hurts if I bend down.[4]
我如果彎下腰就會痛。

Word List ▶▶▶

1 squeeze [skwiz] v. 擠；壓
2 pressure [ˋprɛʃə] n. 壓力

3 crush [krʌʃ] v. 輾壓
4 bend [bɛnd] down 彎腰

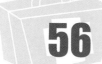

56 咳嗽／呼吸問題──醫護人員詢問

☐ **Can you describe¹ your cough?**

可不可以描述一下你咳嗽的情形？

☐ **Have you ever been diagnosed² with asthma?³**

你是否曾被診斷過有氣喘？

☐ **Are you wheezing⁴ when you breathe?**

你呼吸的時候會有喘聲嗎？

☐ **When do you usually feel shortness of breath?⁵**

你通常什麼時候會覺得喘不過氣來？

☐ **Do you smoke?**

你抽不抽煙？

☐ **Do you find it hard to breathe when you're lying down?**

你平躺的時候是不是會覺得呼吸困難？

Word List ▶ ▶ ▶

1 describe [dɪˋskraɪb] v. 描述
2 diagnose [ˋdaɪəgnoz] v. 診斷
3 asthma [ˋæzmə] n. 氣喘

4 wheeze [hwiz] v. 發出氣喘聲
5 shortness of breath 喘不過氣

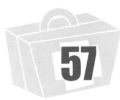

57 咳嗽／呼吸問題——你可以這樣回答

☐ I keep getting this hacking cough.[1]

我一直不斷短促地乾咳。

☐ I'm worried about my shallow breathing.[2]

我對於我的呼吸短促感到有點擔心。

☐ Whenever I breathe in, I can feel a tightness[3] in my chest.

每次吸氣的時候我都覺得胸口緊緊的。

☐ Yes. I smoke a pack a day.

有。我一天抽一包菸。

☐ I can't seem to breathe when I lie on my side.

我側躺的時候似乎無法呼吸。

☐ I cough so much that I start to gag.[4]

我咳嗽得很厲害，咳到會想吐。

5
診療第一步

Word List ▶ ▶ ▶

1 hacking [ˈhækɪŋ] cough 短促頻繁地乾咳

2 shallow [ˈʃælo] breathing 呼吸短淺

3 tightness [ˈtaɪtnɪs] n. 緊密

4 gag [gæg] v. 作嘔；嗆住

58 感染性疾病——醫護人員詢問

☐ **Have you come into contact[1] with any livestock[2] lately?**
你最近是不是有接觸過家畜？

☐ **Have you traveled anywhere recently?**
你最近有沒有去哪裡旅行？

☐ **What vaccines[3] have you received?**
你注射過什麼疫苗？

☐ **Have you been bitten by any insects in the past few days?**
你過去幾天有沒有被蚊蟲叮咬過？

☐ **Have you been having unprotected sex?[4]**
你是不是在從事性行為的時後都沒有做好防預措施？

☐ **I'm putting you on home quarantine[5] for a week.**
我要你做居家隔離一個禮拜。

Word List ▶▶▶

1 contact [`kɑntækt] *n.* 接觸
2 livestock [`laɪv͵stɑk] *n.* 家畜
3 vaccine [`væksin] *n.* 痘苗；疫苗

4 unprotected sex [͵ʌnprəˋtɛktɪd ˋsɛks] *n.* 沒有防護措施的性行為
5 quarantine [`kwɔrən͵tin] *n.* 隔離（home quarantine 指居家隔離）

59 感染性疾病——你可以這樣回答

☐ I've been wearing a facemask[1] all week so I won't infect anyone.

我一整個禮拜都戴著口罩，所以我不會傳染給其他人。

☐ I've been vaccinated[2] against polio,[3] measles,[4] mumps,[5] rubella,[6] and smallpox.[7]

我注射過小兒麻痺、麻疹、腮腺炎、德國麻疹、和天花的疫苗。

☐ I recently came back from South Africa.

我最近剛從南非回來。

☐ I think that I got a tick bite on my camping trip.

我想我在露營的時候被壁蝨叮到了。

☐ No. I always use condoms.[8]

沒有。我都會戴保險套。

☐ How long will it take to know if I've been infected?

要多久才會知道我是否被感染了？

Word List ▶▶▶

1 facemask [ˈfes͵mæsk] *n.* 面罩

2 vaccinate [ˈvæksṇ͵et] *v.* 種牛痘；注射疫苗；接種疫苗

3 polio [ˈpolɪo] *n.* 小兒麻痺症；脊髓灰質炎

4 measles [ˈmizḷz] *n.* 麻疹

5 mumps [mʌmps] *n.* 腮腺炎

6 rubella [ruˋbɛlə] *n.* 德國麻疹

7 smallpox [ˈsmɔl͵pɑks] *n.* 天花

8 condom [ˈkɑndəm] *n.* 保險套

5
診療第一步

60 過敏——醫護人員詢問

☐ Are you allergic¹ to any medication?
你是否對任何藥物過敏？

☐ It looks like allergy season² is here.
看來過敏發生的季節來臨了。

☐ Do you have any pets at home?
你家中是不是有飼養寵物？

☐ Do your allergy symptoms occur³ indoors or outdoors?
你的過敏症狀發生在室內或戶外？

☐ Do any foods cause an allergic reaction?
是不是任何食物都會引起過敏反應？

☐ What are your usual symptoms?
一般你會出現什麼症狀？

Word List ▶▶▶

1 allergic [ə`lɜdʒɪk] *adj.* 過敏的
2 allergy season [`ælədʒɪ͵ sizn] *n.* 過敏發生
的季節

3 occur [ə`kɜ] *v.* 發生

61 過敏——你可以這樣回答

☐ I'm allergic to all types of penicillin.[1]

我對所有的盤尼西林都過敏。

☐ My allergies are out of control.[2] I can't stop sneezing and my eyes are really watery.

我的過敏無法控制。我不斷打噴嚏,而且眼睛一直流眼淚。

☐ I have a dog at home, but I don't seem to be allergic to him.

我家裡養了一隻狗,但是我並不會對牠過敏。

☐ I usually get allergies in spring.

我一到春天就會過敏。

☐ I think I'm allergic to dairy[3] products.

我想我對乳製品過敏。

☐ I have a runny[4] nose first thing in the morning, but it usually clears up by lunchtime.

我早上一起床就會流鼻水,但是到了午餐時間通常就好了。

Word List ▶ ▶ ▶

1 penicillin [ˌpɛnɪˈsɪlɪn] *n.* 盤尼西林

2 out of control 無法控制

3 dairy [ˈdɛrɪ] *adj.* 酪農的;乳酪的(dairy products 指乳製品)

4 runny [ˈrʌnɪ] *adj.* 流鼻涕的

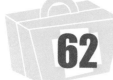
62 皮膚問題——醫護人員詢問

☐ It looks like you have eczema.[1]

看起來你得了濕疹。

☐ When did you first notice these bumps?

你什麼時候第一次注意到這些硬塊？

☐ When did your mole[2] start looking irregular?[3]

你的痣什麼時候開始呈現不規則的形狀？

☐ Is the wart[4] causing you any discomfort?[5]

這個腫瘤有沒有引起你任何的不舒適？

☐ Changing out of sweaty[6] clothes will help keep that jock itch[7] at bay.[8]

換下被汗水濕透的衣物可遠離股癬。

☐ Have you been using any new products on your skin?

你最近有沒有在你的皮膚上塗抹任何新產品？

Word List ▶▶▶

1 eczema [ˋɛksɪmə] *n.* 濕疹

2 mole [mol] *n.* 痣

3 irregular [ɪˋrɛgjələ] *adj.* 不規則狀的

4 wart [wɔrt] *n.* 疣；腫瘤

5 discomfort [dɪsˋkʌmfət] *n.* 不適；不舒服

6 sweaty [ˋswɛtɪ] *adj.* 汗水淋漓的

7 jock itch [ˋdʒɑk ˏɪtʃ] *n.* 股癬；胯下癢

8 keep sth. at bay 使某物不能接近；遏制某物

63 皮膚問題——你可以這樣回答

☐ I have really dry, scaly[1] skin.

我的皮膚非常乾燥，很容易脫皮。

☐ The bumps started appearing two days ago.

這些硬塊在兩天前開始出現。

☐ This mole has gotten a lot bigger and it looks a bit discolored.[2]

這顆痣愈長愈大，而且看起來顏色有一點變。

☐ Does it look cancerous?[3]

是不是看起像癌腫？

☐ The wart doesn't hurt, but can it be removed?

這腫瘤並不會痛，但是可不可以將它切除？

☐ I started using a new moisturizer[4] last week.

我上禮拜開始使用新買的保濕乳液。

5

診療第一步

Word List ▶▶▶

1 scaly [ˈskelɪ] *adj.* 鱗片般剝落的

2 discolored [dɪsˈkʌləd] *v.* 褪色的；變色的

3 cancerous [ˈkænsərəs] *adj.* 癌腫的

4 moisturizer [ˈmɔɪstʃəˌraɪzə] *n.* 潤膚乳液（或霜、露）

醫病診療 900 句典   73

64 足部問題——醫護人員詢問

☐ I can try freezing[1] your wart off. If that doesn't work, you may want to consider surgery.[2]

我可以試著將你的腫瘤凍死掉。如果沒有效，你或許就要考慮動手術。

☐ Does it hurt in the heel or the arch[3] of your foot?

是腳後跟還是你的腳掌內側在痛？

☐ Your toenails[4] can get a fungal[5] infection if you don't change your socks enough, or if you walk barefoot[6] in warm, wet areas.

如果你沒有經常替換襪子，或者在溫暖潮濕的地方光著腳走路，你的腳趾可能會感染黴菌。

☐ Keep your feet dry and use a medicated[7] food powder. That should take care of any foot odors.[8]

腳要保持乾燥，並使用足用藥粉。這樣應該可以解決所有腳臭的問題。

☐ Your foot pain might be due to a condition[9] called flat feet.

你的腳痛應該是一種稱為扁平足的症狀所引起的。

☐ I think your bunions[10] might be caused by your shoes. They look like they're too small for you.

我想你的拇囊腫應該是鞋子造成的。你穿的鞋子看起來太小了。

Word List ▶▶▶

1 freeze [friz] v. 冷凍；凍結
2 surgery [ˋsɝdʒərɪ] n. 外科手術
3 arch [ɑrtʃ] n. 腳掌內側的穹窿
4 toenails [ˋtoˏnelz] n. 腳指甲
5 fungal [ˋfʌŋgl] n. 黴菌的

6 barefoot [ˋbɛrˏfʊt] adv. 赤腳地
7 medicated [ˋmɛdɪˏketɪd] adj. 摻入藥物的
8 odor [ˋodə] n. 氣味
9 condition [kənˋdɪʃən] n. 病症，症狀
10 bunion [ˋbʌnjən] n. 拇囊腫

65 足部問題——你可以這樣問

☐ How did I get corns[1] on top of my toes?
我的腳趾頭頂端為什麼會長雞眼？

☐ I think I may have an ingrown[2] toenail. My big toe is really swollen.
我想我的腳趾甲可能往肉中長了。我的大拇趾腫得很大。

☐ What kind of shoes provides the best support?
什麼樣的鞋子支撐力最好？

☐ I can't seem to get rid of this athlete's foot.[3]
我香港腳的毛病似乎一直好不了。

☐ My toes always seem bent. Is this hammer toe?[4]
我的腳趾看起來總是彎彎的。這是不是槌狀趾？

☐ I think the problem is with my Achilles tendon.[5]
我想這個問題和我的跟腱有關。

Word List ▶▶▶

1 corns [kɔrn] n. 雞眼
2 ingrown [ˋɪnˏgron] adj. 向內生長的；（腳指甲）往肉中生長的
3 athlete's [ˋæθlits] foot n. 香港腳
4 hammer toe [ˋhæməˏto] n. 槌狀趾
5 Achilles tendon [əˋkɪliz ˋtɛndən] n. 跟腱

66 睡眠障礙──醫護人員詢問

☐ **How long have you been having nightmares?**[1]
你作惡夢有多久了？

☐ **How long does it take you to fall asleep?**
你要多久才能入睡？

☐ **What's your bedtime routine?**[2]
你睡前的作息如何？

☐ **Do you feel well rested in the morning?**
你早上起床時是否覺得獲得了充分的休息？

☐ **Do you snore?**[3]
你會不會打鼾？

☐ **Do you wake up in the middle of the night?**
你半夜是不是會醒來？

Word List ▸▸▸

1 nightmare [ˋnaɪt͵mɛr] *n.* 惡夢；夢魘
2 routine [ruˋtin] *n.* 例行公事；常規

3 snore [snor] *v.* 打鼾

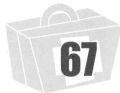

67 睡眠障礙——你可以這樣回答

☐ I toss and turn[1] all night.

我整晚翻來覆去睡不著。

☐ I'm so tired I'm willing to try sleeping pills.[2]

我真的很疲憊，我願意試試安眠藥。

☐ I get about six hours sleep a night.

我晚上大概睡六個小時。

☐ My wife says I keep her awake with all the noise I make.

我太太說我的鼾聲讓她睡不著覺。

☐ I always oversleep.[3]

我總是睡過頭。

☐ I wake up at least two or three times a night to use the bathroom.

我晚上會醒來去上廁所至少兩次或三次。

Word List ▶▶▶

1 toss and turn 輾轉反側
2 sleeping pills 安眠藥

3 oversleep [ˌovəˈslip] v. 睡過頭

5

診療第一步

Part 6

診療第二步——
檢驗

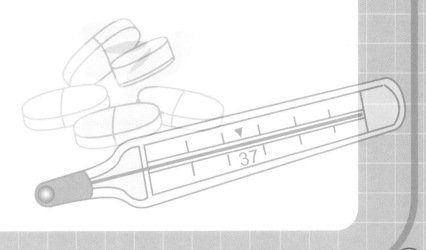

68 醫師的指示 I

☐ (*Looking at your throat*) Open your mouth and say "Ahhhh".

（檢查喉嚨）張開嘴巴，說「阿……」。

☐ (*When listening to your lungs[1]*) Take a deep breath and let it out slowly.

（聆聽你的肺時）深呼吸，然後慢慢吐氣。

☐ (*When taking your blood pressure[2]*) Hold your arm out and try to relax.

（測量你的血壓時）伸出你的手臂，試著放鬆。

☐ (*When taking a blood sample[3]*) Turn your arm out and clench[4] your fist.

（抽驗血液樣本時）把你的手臂轉過來，握緊拳頭。

☐ (*After giving an injection[5]*) Bend your arm and hold this cotton pad[6] in place.

（打完針之後）手臂彎曲，用棉花球按住注射處。

☐ (*Taking your temperature*) Keep the thermometer[7] under your tongue.

（量你的體溫）將體溫計含在你的舌頭下。

Word List ▸ ▸ ▸

1 lung [lʌŋ] *n.* 肺

2 blood pressure 血壓

3 blood sample 血液樣本

4 clench [klɛntʃ] *v.* 握緊

5 injection [ɪn`dʒɛkʃən] *n.* 注射

6 cotton pad 棉花球

7 thermometer [θə`mɑmətə] *n.* 溫度計

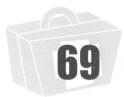

69 醫師的指示 II

☐ Try to raise your arms in the air.

試試把你的雙手舉到空中。

☐ Please lie down on the examination[1] table.

請躺在檢驗台。

☐ Please put on this gown.[2]

請穿上這件長袍。

☐ Turn your head to the (left / right).

把你的頭轉到左邊／右邊。

☐ Follow my finger with your eyes, but don't move your head.

眼睛隨著我的手指移動，但是頭不要動。

☐ I'm going to tap[3] your knee to test your reflexes.[4]

我要輕敲你的膝蓋以測試你的反射神經。

6

診療第二步

Word List ▸▸▸

1 examination [ɪgˌzæməˋneʃən] *n.* 檢查

2 gown [gaʊn] *n.* 袍子

3 tap [tæp] *v.* 輕拍；輕敲

4 reflexes [ˋriflɛksɪz] *n.* 反映；反射作用

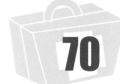

70 對過程提出疑問 I

☐ Will this hurt?

這會痛嗎？

☐ How long do I have to stay in this position?

這個姿勢我要維持多久？

☐ What does my blood pressure reading[1] mean?

我的血壓讀數意味什麼？

☐ Is this really necessary?

這真有必要嗎？

☐ Are there any side effects[2] to this injection?

打這種針是否會引起任何副作用？

☐ Is my temperature considered high?

我的體溫算高嗎？

Word List ▸▸▸

1 reading [ˋridɪŋ] *n.* 讀數（指示的讀數）　　2 side effects 副作用

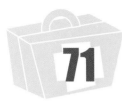

71 對過程提出疑問 II

☐ Do you know what's wrong with me?
你知不知道我的問題出在哪裡？

☐ Is it bad that I can't turn my head?
我的頭不能轉動，這樣是不是很糟？

☐ Is it serious?
是不是很嚴重？

☐ How long is this going to take?
這將會花多少時間？

☐ How often should I get my cholesterol[1] level[2] tested?
我應該多久檢驗一次膽固醇指數？

☐ Ouch! Is it supposed[3] to hurt?
唉喲！這是不是本來就會痛？

Word List ▶ ▶ ▶

1 cholesterol [kə`lɛstə,rol] n. 膽固醇
2 level [`lɛvl] n. 程度；層次

3 supposed [sə`pozd] adj. 被認為應當的

Part 7

癒後和治療

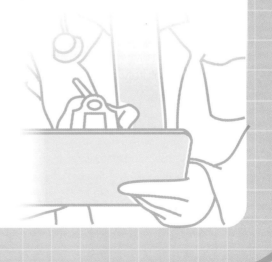

72 你很好

☐ You're going to be fine.
你不會有問題的。

☐ It looks like it cleared up on its own.
看來它自行消失了。

☐ You're in the clear.[1]
你已經沒問題了。

☐ You have nothing to worry about.
你沒什麼好擔心的。

☐ I think I can give you a clean bill of health.[2]
我想我可以確認你的健康狀況良好。

☐ There's absolutely nothing wrong with you. Except maybe hypochondria.[3]
你一點問題也沒有——除了可能得了憂鬱症。

Word List ▶ ▶ ▶

1 in the clear 病症解除

2 give sb. a clean bill of health 確認某人的健康狀況良好

3 hypochondria [ˌhaɪpəˋkɑndrɪə] *n.* 憂鬱症

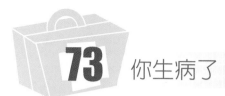

73 你生病了

☐ You've got a mild case of tonsillitis.[1]
你得了輕微的扁桃腺炎。

☐ It's a good thing you came in.
還好你有來看病。

☐ We're going to have to run some more tests.
我們還要多做一些檢驗。

☐ I'm going to send you to a specialist.[2]
我要將你轉給專科醫生。

☐ You're suffering[3] from dehydration.[4]
你顯現出的病狀是脫水。

☐ I'm afraid it's more serious than we thought.
恐怕比我們先前想的還要嚴重。

Word List ▶▶▶

1 tonsillitis [ˌtɑnslˈaɪtɪs] *n.* 扁桃腺炎

2 specialist [ˈspɛʃəlɪst] *n.* 專科醫生

3 suffer [ˈsʌfɚ] *v.* 患病

4 dehydration [ˌdihaɪˈdreʃən] *n.* 脫水

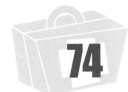

74 用藥和處方

☐ Take this prescription[1] to a pharmacy[2] and have it filled[3] right away.
立刻拿這個處方到藥局去，請他們依處方給藥。

☐ This medicine will help fight the infection.
這個藥方有助於對抗感染。

☐ Remember to finish the entire course of antibiotics.[4]
記得要把整個療程的抗生素服用完畢。

☐ Take this before bedtime if you have trouble sleeping.
如果你有睡眠障礙，睡前服用這個藥。

☐ You can stop taking this tablet[5] as soon as you feel better.
你只要覺得好轉，就可以停止服用這種藥片。

☐ This medication should be taken on an empty stomach.
這種藥應該空腹吃。

Word List ▶▶▶

1 prescription [prɪˋskrɪpʃən] *n.* 處方；藥方
2 pharmacy [ˋfɑrməsɪ] *n.* 藥房
3 fill [fɪl] *v.* 配（藥）

4 antibiotic [͵æntɪbaɪˋɑtɪk] *n.* 抗生素
5 tablet [ˋtæblɪt] *n.* 藥片

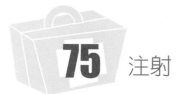

75 注射

☐ We'll have to give you a shot for your allergic reaction.

我們得幫你注射過敏反應的針。

☐ You'll feel better once we hook you up to an IV.[1]

只要我們幫你打點滴，你就會覺得比較舒服。

☐ It's been a while since your last immunization.[2] You're going to need a booster shot.[3]

距離你上次打預防針已經有一段時間了。你必須施打加強針。

☐ This injection will cause some swelling, but it should go down in a few days.

這次的注射會有點腫，但是過幾天應該就會消了。

☐ Don't worry. It's just like a pinprick.[4]

不用擔心，就像被針扎一下。

☐ An injection is the most effective way to get the medicine into your bloodstream.[5]

打針是讓藥劑進入血脈內最有效的方法。

Word List ▶ ▶ ▶

1 IV= intravenous [ˌɪntrəˈvinəs] n. 靜脈注射 （即點滴）

2 immunization [ˌɪmjʊnəˈzeʃən] n. （免疫） 預防針

3 booster shot [ˈbustə] n. 加強針（後續的疫苗注射）

4 pinprick [ˈpɪnˌprɪk] n. 針刺

5 bloodstream [ˈblʌdˌstrim] n. 體內血液的流動

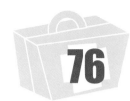

76 藥瓶上的標示 I

(Part I)

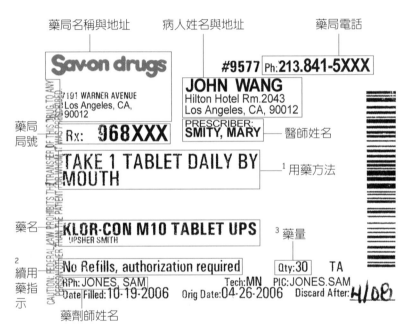

藥局名稱與地址　　病人姓名與地址　　　藥局電話

藥局局號

醫師姓名

1 用藥方法

藥名

2 續用藥指示

藥劑師姓名

3 藥量

Sav-on drugs

7191 WARNER AVENUE
Los Angeles, CA,
90012

Rx: **968XXX**

TAKE 1 TABLET DAILY BY MOUTH

KLOR-CON M10 TABLET UPS
UPSHER SMITH

No Refills, authorization required

RPh: JONES, SAM
Date Filled: 10-19-2006

CAUTION: FEDERAL LAW PROHIBITS THE TRANSFER OF THIS DRUG TO ANY PERSON OTHER THAN THE PATIENT FOR WHOM IT WAS PRESCRIBED

#9577 Ph: 213.841-5XXX

JOHN WANG
Hilton Hotel Rm.2043
Los Angeles, CA, 90012

PRESCRIBER:
SMITY, MARY

Qty: 30   TA

Tech: MN   PIC: JONES.SAM
Orig Date: 04-26-2006   Discard After: 4/08

1 用藥方法：Take 1 tablet daily by mouth 每日口服一個藥片

2 續用藥指示：No refills, authorization required 不可續藥，需要醫師指示

3 藥量：Qty = Quality

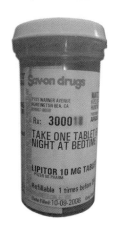

(Part II) 服藥指示

MAY DISSOLVE IN WATER. STIR-SWALLOW. RINSE DOWN W/WATER. DO NOT CHEW PIECES —— ① 可溶解在水裡。攪拌後吞服。
跟水一起服下 (W / WATER)。
不可嚼碎。

TAKE THIS MEDICATION WITH PLENTY OF WATER. —— ② 服藥需配大量的水

TAKE WITH FOOD —— ③ 可與食物同時服用

TAKE OR USE THIS EXACTLY AS DIRECTED. DO NOT SKIP DOSES OR DISCONTINUE. —— ④ 依照指示服用。不可斷斷續續或停用。

This is a(n) WHITE, OBLONG-shaped TAB imprinted with KC M10 on the front. —— ⑤ 這是白色、橢圓形的藥片，印有 KC M10 字樣在上面

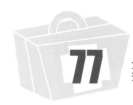

77 藥瓶上的標示 II

(Part I)

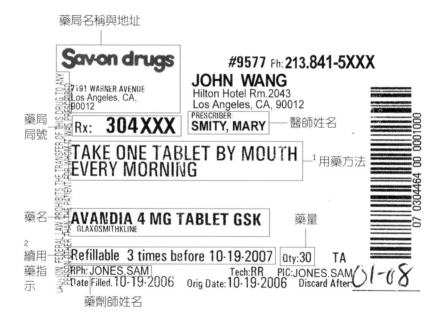

藥局名稱與地址

Sav-on drugs

7191 WARNER AVENUE
Los Angeles, CA,
90012

#9577 Fh:**213.841-5XXX**

JOHN WANG
Hilton Hotel Rm.2043
Los Angeles, CA, 90012

PRESCRIBER:
SMITY, MARY ——醫師姓名

藥局
局號   Rx: **304XXX**

**TAKE ONE TABLET BY MOUTH
EVERY MORNING** ——¹ 用藥方法

藥名   **AVANDIA 4 MG TABLET GSK**   藥量
       GLAXOSMITHKLINE

2
續用   **Refillable 3 times before 10-19-2007**   Qty:30   TA
藥指   RPh:JONES.SAM   Tech:RR   PIC:JONES.SAM
示   Date Filled:10-19-2006   Orig Date:10-19-2006   Discard After:**01-08**
       藥劑師姓名

CAUTION FEDERAL LAW PROHIBITS THE TRANSFER OF THIS DRUG TO ANY PERSON OTHER THAN THE PATIENT FOR WHOM IT WAS PRESCRIBED

1 用藥方法：Take one tablet by mouth every morning 每日早上口服一個藥片
2 續用藥指示：Refillable 3 times before 10-19-2007 可續藥三次，至 2007 年
   10 月 19 日之前為止

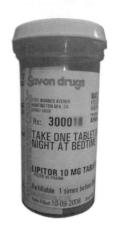

(Part II) 服藥指示

This is a(n) ORANGE, PENTAGON-shaped TABLET imprinted with 4 on the front and SB on the back.

① 這是橘色、五角形藥片，正面印有 4，反面印有 SB 字樣。

DO NOT USE IF PREGNANT OR SUSPECT YOU ARE PREGNANT OR ARE BREAST FEEDING.

② 懷孕者、或是疑似有受孕，或是哺乳者不可使用。

THIS MEDICATION MAY BE TAKEN WITH OR WITHOUT FOOD.

③ 可與食物或不與食物同時服用

Don't Wait, Call A Day Ahead

④ 依照指示服用。不可斷斷續續或停用。

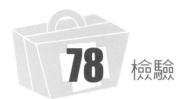
78 檢驗

☐ I'd like to schedule[1] you for an MRI.[2]

我要為你安排時間進行核磁共振檢驗。

☐ I'm going to draw some blood[3] today and send it to the lab. We should get the results back on Thursday.

我今天要抽一點血並送到實驗室。我們星期四就應該可以知道結果了。

☐ The EKG[4] confirmed our initial[5] diagnosis.[6]

心電圖證實我們初步的診斷無誤。

☐ The results were inconclusive.[7]

從報告結果無法做出結論。

☐ The test came back positive[8] / negative.[9]

檢驗結果呈現陽性／陰性。

☐ Your urine test showed a high level of uric acid,[10] which is what causes kidney[11] stones.

你的尿液檢驗顯示尿酸指數很高，這是引起腎結石的原因。

Word List ▶▶▶

1 schedule [ˋskɛdʒʊl] v. 安排時間
2 MRI = Magnetic Resonance Imaging [mægˋnɛtɪk ˋrɛzṇəns ˋɪmɪdʒɪŋ] 核磁共振造影
3 draw blood 抽血
4 EKG = electrocardiogram [ɪˋlɛktroˋkɑrdɪəˏgræm] n. 心電圖

5 initial [ɪˋnɪʃəl] adj. 最初的
6 diagnosis [ˏdaɪəgˋnosɪs] n. 診斷
7 inconclusive [ˏɪnkənˋklusɪv] adj. 未獲結論的；未確定的
8 positive [ˋpɑzətɪv] adj. 陽性的
9 negative [ˋnɛgətɪv] adj. 陰性的
10 uric acid [ˋjʊrɪk ˋæsɪd] n. 尿酸
11 kidney stone [ˋkɪdnɪˏston] n. 腎結石

79 手術

☐ We may have to consider surgery.
我們或許必須考慮動手術。

☐ Surgery is your only option.[1]
手術是你唯一的選擇。

☐ It's a minor operation,[2] but there are some risks.[3]
這是個小手術，但是有些風險。

☐ Recovery[4] time would take at least four weeks.
要復元至少需要四個禮拜的時間。

☐ It's a very routine[5] surgery. We usually do it on an outpatient[6] basis.
這只是例行性手術。我們通常會對門診病人進行這類手術。

☐ We will monitor[7] your situation and see if surgery is the way to go.
我們會追蹤你的情況，看看是否有動手術的必要。

Word List ▶▶▶

1 option [ˈɑpʃən] n. 選擇
2 minor operation [ˈmaɪnəˌɑpəˈreʃən] n. 小型手術
3 risk [rɪsk] n. 風險
4 recovery [rɪˈkʌvərɪ] n. 復元；康復
5 routine [ruˈtin] adj. 例行的
6 outpatient [ˈaʊtˌpeʃənt] n. 門診病人
7 monitor [ˈmɑnətə] v. 監聽；監測；監視

80 關於飲食的建議

☐ Cut out all foods containing gluten.[1]
所有含有麵筋的食物都不要吃。

☐ You need to cut down on your sodium[2] intake.[3]
你必須減少鈉的攝取。

☐ Pay attention to how much fat you consume[4] each day.
留意你每天脂肪的攝取量。

☐ You should get on a high-protein[5] diet.
你應該進行高蛋白飲食食療法。

☐ Avoid all refined sugars[6] and carbohydrates.[7]
避免攝取任何精製糖和碳水化合物。

☐ Make sure you get enough fiber.[8]
一定要攝取足夠的纖維。

Word List ▸▸▸

1 gluten [ˋɡlutən] *n.* 穀蛋白黏膠質（即麵筋）
2 sodium [ˋsodɪəm] *n.* 鈉
3 intake [ˋɪn͵tek] *n.* 吸收
4 consume [kənˋsum] *v.* 消耗；吃、喝

5 high-protein [ˋhaɪˋprotiɪn] *adj.* 高蛋白質的
6 refined sugar [rɪˋfaɪndˋʃʊgɚ] *n.* 精製糖
7 carbohydrate [͵kɑrboˋhaɪdret] *n.* 碳水化合物
8 fiber [ˋfaɪbɚ] *n.* 纖維

81 關於飲食的疑問

☐ Am I allowed to eat dairy products?

我可以吃乳製品嗎?

☐ Can I still drink beer?

我還可以喝啤酒嗎?

☐ (*Pointing to a food list*) Are these foods completely off-limits,[1] or am I allowed them in moderation?[2]

(手比著食物清單) 這些食物是不是完全禁止,還是我可以適量地攝取?

☐ If I limit these foods, will I still get enough calcium?[3]

如果我禁吃這些食物,我鈣的攝取量是否還會足夠?

☐ What kind of vitamins should I be taking? Is a daily multivitamin[4] enough?

我應該吃哪種維他命?一天一顆綜合維他命夠不夠?

☐ How can I maintain a well-balanced[5] diet?

我要如何才能維持均衡的飲食?

Word List ▶▶▶

1 off-limits [`ɔf`lɪmɪts] *adj.* 禁止進入的
2 moderation [ˌmɑdə`reʃən] *n.* 節制;適度
3 calcium [`kælsɪəm] *n.* 鈣

4 multivitamin [ˌmʌltə`vaɪtəmɪn] *n.* 綜合維他命
5 well-balanced [`wɛl`bælənst] *adj.* 均衡的

82 其他建議

☐ Rest up. Don't do anything too strenuous[1] this week.
多休息。這個禮拜不要做太費力的工作。

☐ You should do at least 30 minutes of exercise everyday.
你每天應該至少運動三十分鐘。

☐ Try to get seven to eight hours of sleep each night.
每天晚上試著睡七到八小時。

☐ Drink plenty of fluids.[2] Water and tea are best.
多喝流質。最好是喝水和茶。

☐ Stick to bland[3] food for the next few days.
未來這幾天飲食要保持清淡。

☐ If you don't feel better in a week, come see me again.
如果一個禮拜後還是不舒服，再回來看診。

Word List ▸▸▸

1 strenuous [ˈstrɛnjʊəs] *adj.* 費力的
2 fluid [ˈfluɪd] *n.* 流質；液態物

3 bland [blænd] *adj.* 溫和的；無刺激性的

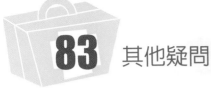

83 其他疑問

☐ I have a business trip the day after tomorrow. Can I still go?

我後天要出差。我還可不可以去？

☐ Will I still be able to fly?

我還可不可以坐飛機？

☐ What kind of exercise do you recommend?[1]

你建議做什麼樣的運動？

☐ Should I wait for this to completely clear up before returning to work?

我是不是應該等完全復原之後再回去工作？

☐ Is there anything I can do to speed up[2] my recovery?

要快一點康復有什麼我可以做的？

☐ How can I make sure I don't give it to anyone else?

我要如何才能確保不會傳染給其他人？

Word List ▸ ▸ ▸

1 recommend [ˌrɛkəˋmɛnd] v. 建議　　　2 speed up 加快速度

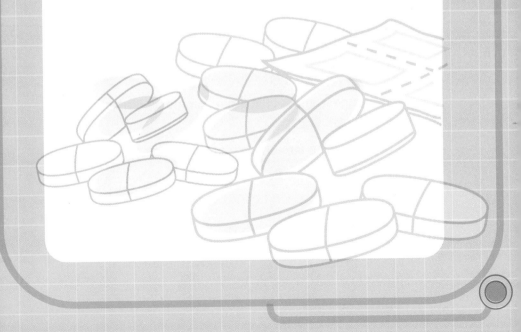

Part **8**

病人的問題與疑慮

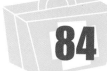

84 對於藥物的疑慮

醫護人員可能這樣說

☐ This pill might make you feel listless.[1]

這種藥丸可能會讓你有倦怠感。

☐ It's not unusual for patients to experience blurred[2] vision at the beginning of treatment.

病人在治療初期出現視線模糊的情形是常有的。

☐ Don't drink alcohol while taking this medication.

服用這種藥物期間不要喝酒。

你可以這樣說

☐ Are there any harmful[3] side effects?

這有沒有什麼有害的副作用？

☐ Is it safe to ingest[4] more than the recommended amount?

服用比建議量還多，安全嗎？

☐ Can I take this if I'm already on blood pressure medication?[5]

如果我已經在服用降血壓的藥，還可以吃這種藥嗎？

Word List ▶▶▶

1 listless [ˋlɪstlɪs] *adj.* 無精打采的；倦怠的

2 blurred [blɜd] *adj.* 模糊不清的

3 alcohol [ˋælkəˌhɔl] *n.* 酒精；酒

4 harmful [ˋhɑrmfəl] *adj.* 有害的

5 ingest [ɪnˋdʒɛst] *v.* 攝取

6 medication [ˌmɛdɪˋkeʃən] *n.* 藥物；藥物治療

MP3 ▶▶ 085

85 詢問醫生的專業背景

☐ Have you performed[1] this procedure[2] before?

你以前動過這種手術嗎？

☐ How many people have you diagnosed[3] with this condition?

你以前診斷過多少人有這種症狀？

☐ Do you have a lot of experience in this area?

你這個領域方面的經驗很豐富嗎？

☐ Where did you receive your training?[4]

你在哪裡受的訓練？

☐ Have you ever seen something like this before?

你以前看過類似的例子嗎？

☐ Are you up to date[5] with new developments in treating this illness?

你知不知道治療這種疾病的最新方法？

Word List ▶▶▶

1 perform [pɚˋfɔrm] v. 履行；執行、完成

2 procedure [prəˋsidʒɚ] n. 程序；手術

3 diagnose [ˋdaɪəgnoz] v. 診斷

4 training [ˋtrenɪŋ] n. 訓練

5 up to date 保持不落後

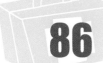

86 諮詢專家或詢問其他意見

☐ I think I'd like to get a second opinion.[1]
我想我要徵詢其他意見。

☐ Is there any way to double-check?[2]
有沒有方法可以做再確認？

☐ I'd prefer to see a few more doctors before making a decision.
我想多看幾位醫生再做決定。

☐ Can you recommend a qualified[3] specialist?
你可不可以推薦一位合格的專科醫師？

☐ Who should I see to get a better picture[4] of what I'm facing?
我應該看哪一位醫師才會比較了解我目前面臨的狀況？

☐ Thank you for your time, but I'd be more comfortable seeing another doctor or two.
佔用了你的時間，謝謝，但是再多看一、兩位醫生我會覺得比較安心。

Word List ▶ ▶ ▶

1 a second opinion 其他的意見
2 double-check [ˋdʌbl̩ˏtʃɛk] v. 仔細檢查；進行復核
3 qualified [ˋkwɑləˏfaɪd] adj. 合格的
4 get a better picture 對狀況情形更加了解

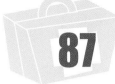

87 諮詢醫療建議

☐ Is this procedure safe?
做這個安不安全？

☐ What's the success rate of this treatment?
這種療法成功機率有多高？

☐ Is this the newest treatment available?
這是不是目前能做最新的療法？

☐ What are my other options?
還有其他選擇嗎？

☐ In your professional[1] opinion, which treatment is best suited[2] for my situation?
依你專業的角度看，哪一種療法最適合我的狀況？

☐ What would happen if I didn't do anything?
如果我不採取任何行動結果會如何？

Word List ▶ ▶ ▶

1 professional [prə`fɛʃən!] *adj.* 職業的；專業的
2 suited [`sutɪd] *adj.* 合適的

Part 9

住院

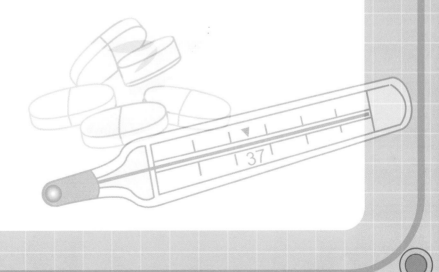

88 詢問病房

你可以這樣問

☐ How much is a private[1] room?
單人房的價格是多少？

☐ How many people are there in a shared[2] room?
多人房住幾個人？

☐ Can my husband / wife stay in the room with me?
我先生／太太可不可以待在房裡陪我？

醫護人員可能這樣回答

☐ We have private, shared, and group rooms. Which would you prefer?
我們有單人、多人以及團體病房。你想要哪一種？

☐ It's two people to a room.
兩個人住一間。

☐ Of course. We can put a cot[3] in your room for your spouse.[4]
當然可以。我們可以放一張便床給你的配偶。

Word List ▸▸▸

1 private [ˋpraɪvɪt] *adj.* 私人的；個人的
2 shared [ʃɛrd] *adj.* 分享的

3 cot [kɑt] *n.* （摺疊式）便床
4 spouse [spauz] *n.* 配偶

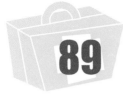

89 住院細節

你可以這樣問

☐ When are visiting hours?
探病時段是什麼時候？

☐ Am I allowed to leave my room whenever I want?
我能不能隨時離開病房？

☐ Where is the cafeteria[1] located?
自助餐廳在哪裡？

醫護人員可能這樣回答

☐ Regular visiting hours are from 9 a.m. to 9 p.m.
一般探病時間是早上九點到晚上九點。

☐ As long as you're mobile,[2] you can walk in the hallway or sit outside.
只要你可以走動，你可以在走廊散散步或到外面坐坐。

☐ The hospital has a cafeteria, coffee shop, gift shop, pharmacy, and chapel.[3]
醫院設有自助餐廳、咖啡廳、禮品店、藥局和教堂。

Word List ▶▶▶

1 cafeteria [ˌkæfəˈtɪrɪə] n. 自助餐館
2 mobile [ˈmobl̩] adj. 可動的；流動性的

3 chapel [ˈtʃæpl̩] n.（學校、醫院、軍營等的）附屬禮拜堂

90 住院的請求

☐ Is there a choice of meals?
用餐有沒有選擇？

☐ Can I get an extra pillow, please?
麻煩你，我可不可以多要一個枕頭？

☐ Is it possible to turn down the air conditioner?[1]
有沒有可能把冷氣溫度調低一點？

☐ I think I may need help getting to the bathroom.
我想我可能需要人扶我進洗手間。

☐ What should I do if I need assistance?[2]
假如我需要協助該怎麼辦？

☐ Can you give me anything to help me sleep?
你可不可以開些藥給我好幫助我入睡？

Word List ▶ ▶ ▶

1 air conditioner [ˈɛr kənˌdɪʃənə] n.
冷氣機
2 assistance [əˈsɪstəns] n. 協助；幫助

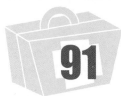

91 醫護人員的回應

☐ Do you need another blanket[1] as well?

你是不是也需要多一張毯子？

☐ The thermostat[2] is right by the light switch.

自動調溫器就在電燈開關的右邊。

☐ If you need anything, just push the call button[3] next to your bed.

如果你需要任何東西，只要按下床邊的呼叫按鈕就行了。

☐ If there's an emergency,[4] push this red button.

如果有緊急狀況，按下這個紅色按鈕。

☐ If you want to go to the bathroom, you have to wheel[5] your IV drip[6] in with you.

你如果想上洗手間，必須把你的點滴一起推進去。

☐ I'm sorry, there's no TV in shared rooms after ten o'clock.

對不起，多人房在十點之後不能看電視。

Word List ▶▶▶

1 blanket [`blæŋkɪt] n. 毯子；毛毯

2 thermostat [`θɜmə,stæt] n. 自動調溫器；恆溫器

3 call button [`kɔl,bʌtn̩] n. 呼叫按鈕

4 emergency [ɪ`mɝdʒənsɪ] n. 緊急情況

5 wheel [hwil] v. 轉動；滾動

6 drip [drɪp] n. 滴落；滴液（IV drip 即點滴）

Part 10

意外和緊急事件

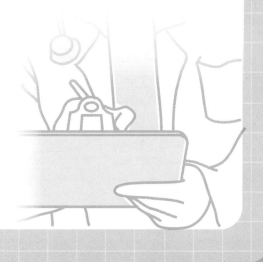

92 打911

☐ I need an ambulance,[1] and quickly!
我需要救護車，快一點！

☐ My friend is having a heart attack.
我的朋友心臟病發作了。

☐ My son fell down and broke his leg.
我兒子跌到，摔斷了腿。

☐ There's a car accident[2] on Highway 9.
九號高速公路上發生了車禍。

☐ Someone fainted[3] and I don't know what to do.
有人昏倒了，我不知道該怎麼辦。

☐ Help, my daughter is choking![4] What should I do?
救命啊！我的女兒噎著了！我該怎麼做？

Word List ▶▶▶

1 ambulance [ˋæmbjələns] *n.* 救護車
2 accident [ˋæksədənt] *n.* 事故；意外事情
3 faint [fent] *v.* 昏厥；暈倒
4 choke [tʃok] *v.* 噎住；塞住；哽住

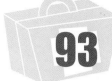

93 911 醫護人員的回應

☐ 美國： 911. What is your emergency?[1]

這裡是 911。您發生了什麼緊急狀況？

英國： Emergency. What service do you require?

這是緊急中心。您需要幫什麼忙？

☐ Please calm down. What is the problem?

請冷靜下來。發生了什麼問題？

☐ Where are you calling from? What's the nearest cross street[2] / intersection?[3]

你的電話是從哪裡打來的？離你最近的交叉口在哪裡？

☐ Who is injured? When did this happen?

誰受傷了？什麼時候發生的？

☐ What is your name? What is your telephone number?

你叫什麼姓名？電話號碼是多少？

☐ Stay on the phone. Don't hang up.[4] An ambulance is coming now.

待在電話旁，別掛斷。救護車馬上就到。

Word List ▶▶▶

1 emergency [ɪˋmɜdʒənsɪ] *n.* 緊急情況；突然事件

2 cross street [ˋkrɔs͵strit] *n.* 十字路口

3 intersection [͵ɪntɚˋsɛkʃən] *n.* 十字路口

4 hang up 掛斷電話

94 911 的指示

☐ Place a blanket[1] over him and wait for the ambulance to arrive.
用一條毯子蓋在他身上,然後等候救護車抵達。

☐ Try to keep her awake and calm.
試著讓她保持清醒、冷靜。

☐ Raise the injured leg and use whatever you can to stop the bleeding.
把受傷的腿抬高,想辦法找東西止血。

☐ Lift up his head and keep him comfortable.
把他的頭抬高,讓他舒服一點。

☐ Give her some water to drink if you have some.
如果有水的話,給她喝一點。

☐ Don't move the victim[2] until the paramedics[3] arrive.
在醫護人員抵達之前,不要移動傷患。

Word List ▶▶▶

1 blanket [ˋblæŋkɪt] *n.* 毯子
2 victim [ˋvɪktɪm] *n.* 受害者;遇難者
3 paramedic [͵pærəˋmɛdɪk] *n.* 醫務輔助人員

95 幫助傷者保持冷靜

☐ Don't worry. Everything is going to be just fine.

不要擔心。不會有事的。

☐ The ambulance is on its way.

救護車已經在路上了。

☐ Help is coming. Just hang in there.[1]

救援馬上就到。請撐住。

☐ I know it hurts, but we'll get you to the hospital.

我知道很痛,我們會送你到醫院的。

☐ Try to relax. Take a few deep breaths.

試著放鬆。深呼吸幾下。

☐ Calm down.[2] We'll take care of you.

冷靜一下,我們會照顧你的。

10

意外和緊急事件

Word List ▶ ▶ ▶

1 hang in there 堅持下去;撐下去   2 Calm down. 冷靜下來。

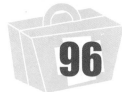

96 指示傷患

☐ **Try to sit up.**[1]
試試坐起來。

☐ **Try not to move.**
儘量不要動。

☐ **Don't talk. Save your strength.**[2]
不要說話，保留你的體力。

☐ **Do you think you can try and walk?**
你可不可以試著走走看？

☐ **How many fingers am I holding up?**
我現在舉起幾根手指？

☐ **Don't fall asleep. Look at me.**
不要睡著。看著我。

Word List ▶▶▶

1 sit up 坐起來

2 strength [strɛŋθ] *n.* 力量；力氣

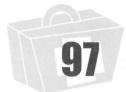

97 指示旁觀者

☐ Someone call 911.
誰可以打電話給 911。

☐ Try not to crowd[1] around him.
儘量不要圍在他身邊。

☐ Give her some room to breathe.
留一點空間讓她呼吸。

☐ Does anyone know CPR?[2]
有沒有人知道怎麼進行心肺復甦術？

☐ Does anyone have something we can cover[3] him up with?
有沒有人有東西可以蓋在他身上？

☐ Someone help me prop her up.[4]
誰可以幫我把她撐起來。

Word List ▶▶▶

1 crowd [kraud] v. 圍住
2 CPR = cardiopulmonary resuscitation
[ˌkɑrdɪoˈpʌlməˌnɛrɪ rɪˌsʌsəˈteʃən] 心肺復甦術

3 cover [ˈkʌvə] v. 覆蓋；遮蓋
4 prop up 支撐；扶持

98 去急診室——醫護人員詢問

☐ Are you a relative?[1]

你是不是親屬？

☐ What's your relationship[2] to the patient?

你和病人是什麼關係？

☐ How did this happen?

這是怎麼發生的？

☐ I'm sorry. You're going to have to wait outside.

對不起，你必須在外面等。

☐ Is she allergic to any medication?

她有沒有對任何藥物過敏？

☐ Please ask his wife to come to the hospital as soon as possible.

請叫他太太儘快到醫院來。

Word List ▶▶▶

1 relative [ˈrɛlətɪv] n. 親屬

2 relationship [rɪˈleʃənˌʃɪp] n. 關係

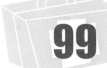
99 去急診室——你可以這麼說

☐ I don't know how it happened.

我不知道是怎麼發生的。

☐ He doesn't have any family here.

他在這裡沒有任何家屬。

☐ When will we find out if she's OK?

我們什麼時候才會知道她有沒有事？

☐ Her husband won't be able to get here until this evening.

她先生今天晚上才趕得到。

☐ How does it look?

狀況看起來如何？

☐ What's happening right now?

現在的情形怎麼樣？

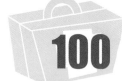

100 骨頭斷裂／骨折 I —— 提問

☐ I was playing racquetball[1] and landed[2] on my arm.
我在打短網拍牆球，不慎手臂著地。

☐ I slipped[3] on a patch of ice.
我在一塊冰地上滑倒了。

☐ Is my ankle broken, or is it just a sprain?[4]
我的腳踝是斷裂了，還是只是扭傷？

☐ Will I need a cast?[5]
我需要上石膏嗎？

☐ How long will I be in a cast for?
我石膏要上多久？

☐ What is a stress fracture?[6]
什麼是壓迫性骨折？

Word List ▶▶▶

1 racquetball [ˋrækɪtˏbɔl] n. 短網拍牆球
2 land [lænd] v. 著陸
3 slip [slɪp] v. 滑倒；失足
4 sprain [spren] n. 扭傷

5 cast [kæst] n. 固定用敷料；石膏
6 stress fracture [ˋstrɛs ˏfræktʃɚ] n. 壓迫性骨折

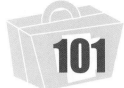

101 骨頭斷裂／骨折 II ── 醫護人員的回應

☐ Your leg will be in a cast for eight weeks.
你的腳需要上八個禮拜的石膏。

☐ You've suffered a really bad break.[1] You'll need surgery.
你骨頭碎裂的情形很嚴重，必須動手術。

☐ We can give you a walking cast[2] to make it easier to move around.
我們可以給你上活動式石膏，讓你的行動比較自如。

☐ Don't get your cast wet. Use a waterproof[3] cover when you take a shower.
你上的石膏不要弄濕了。洗澡時要使用防水套。

☐ We'll have to put a pin[4] in your arm to make sure it sets[5] properly.
我們要在你的手臂上打釘以確保斷骨能癒合。

☐ It looks like you have a dislocated[6] shoulder.[7]
看起來你的肩膀脫臼了。

Word List ▶▶▶

1 break [brek] *n.* 骨折
2 walking cast 活動式石膏
3 waterproof [ˋwɔtɚ͵pruf] *adj.* 防水的；不透水的

4 pin [pɪn] *n.* 別針
5 set [sɛt] *v.* 接合（斷骨），癒合
6 dislocated [ˋdɪsləٜketɪd] *v.* 脫臼的
7 shoulder [ˋʃoldɚ] *n.* 肩膀

102 昏倒 I——描述症狀

☐ I felt a little woozy[1] this morning.
我今天早上覺得頭有點暈。

☐ The last thing I remember was trying to open the door.
我最後記得的事是當時我正要把門打開。

☐ I've had these fainting[2] spells[3] for two weeks now.
我這兩個禮拜以來經常昏倒。

☐ I felt really weak when I came to.
我恢復知覺時覺得非常虛弱。

☐ I stood up really quickly and then lost my balance.
我非常快地站起來，結果失去平衡。

☐ It was really stuffy[4] in the room.
那房間裡非常悶。

Word List ▶▶▶

1 woozy [ˋwuzɪ] *adj.* 頭昏眼花的
2 fainting [ˋfentɪŋ] *adj.* 昏倒的
3 spell [spɛl] *n.* （疾病等的）一陣發作
4 stuffy [ˋstʌfɪ] *adj.* 窒悶的；通風不良的

103 昏倒 II——醫護人員的回應

☐ Has this happened before?

以前有沒有發生過這種情形？

☐ Are you experiencing any other symptoms?[1]

你還有沒有其他任何症狀？

☐ You may have very low blood pressure.

你可能是血壓太低。

☐ I'd like to order a blood test and see if there are any other underlying[2] causes.[3]

我要做血液檢查，看看是否有其他任何潛在的因素。

☐ Are you eating enough?

你的飲食夠不夠量？

☐ Have you been feeling stressed[4] lately?

你最近是不是覺得壓力很大？

Word List ▶ ▶ ▶

1 symptom [ˋsɪmptəm] *n.* 症狀

2 underlying [ˌʌndəˋlaɪɪŋ] *adj.* 潛在性的

3 causes [kɔz] *n.* 原因；起因

4 stressed [strɛst] *adj.* 緊張的；感到有壓力的

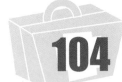

104 脫水 I──描述症狀

☐ I don't know why I didn't feel thirsty.
我不知為什麼都不覺得渴。

☐ I was really parched,[1] but I couldn't find anything to drink.
我簡直要渴死了，但是就是找不到東西喝。

☐ I've been out in the sun all day.
我一整天都在戶外曬太陽。

☐ I may have been overdoing[2] it.
我可能曬過頭了。

☐ I felt a bit lightheaded,[3] but I didn't think it was serious.
我感覺頭有一點暈，但是沒覺得那很嚴重。

☐ I've had the stomach flu[4] and I just can't keep anything down.
我得了急性腸胃炎，吃什麼就吐什麼。

Word List ▶▶▶

1 parch [pɑrtʃ] v. 使乾透；使焦乾

2 overdo [ˌovɚˋdu] v. 做的過分；做的過火

3 lightheaded [ˋlaɪtˋhɛdɪd] adj. 頭暈的

4 stomach flu [ˋstʌmək‚flu] n. 腸胃炎

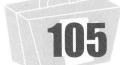

105 脫水 II——醫護人員的回應

☐ Try to drink small amounts of fluids at regular intervals.[1]
試著每隔一段時間喝少量的流質。

☐ Don't drink too much water at once. It might make you vomit.
不要一下子喝太多水，這樣可能會讓你想吐。

☐ Have you had diarrhea[2] lately?
你最近有沒有腹瀉？

☐ Avoid sports drinks. They contain too much sugar.
避免喝運動飲料，裡面糖分太多。

☐ I'm going to put you on an IV.
我要幫你注射點滴。

☐ Try to keep cool. Don't get overheated.[3]
儘量保持清涼，不要熱過頭了。

10

意外和緊急事件

Word List ▶▶▶

1 interval [ˋɪntəvl̩] *n.* 間隔

2 diarrhea [͵daɪəˋriə] *n.* 腹瀉

3 overheated [͵ovəˋhitɪd] *adj.* 過熱的；過度
興奮的

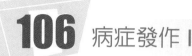

106 病症發作 I ——醫療人員詢問

☐ Have you ever had a seizure[1] before?
你以前有沒有過發作的紀錄？

☐ How long did the episode[2] last for?
發作的時間持續多久？

☐ Do you remember what happened during the seizure?
你記不記得發作的經過？

☐ Have you been diagnosed with epilepsy?[3]
你以前有沒有被診斷出有癲癇症？

☐ Have you experienced any memory loss[4] from the seizure?
你有沒有過因為發作而喪失記憶？

☐ Are you on any medication for your seizures?
你目前是不是正在服用防治發作的藥物？

Word List ▶▶▶

1 seizure [ˋsiʒɚ] *n.* （疾病後）突然發作
2 episode [ˋɛpə͵sod] *n.* （病症的發作的）一回

3 epilepsy [ˋɛpə͵lɛpsɪ] *n.* 癲癇；羊癇瘋
4 memory loss 記憶喪失

107 病症發作 II ——你可以這麼說

MP3 ▸▸ 107

□ I had a seizure a few years ago, but nothing since then.
我幾年前有過發作的紀錄，但之後都沒再發過。

□ I don't usually remember my seizures, but this time, I was conscious[1] while it was happening.
我發作時通常什麼都不記得，但是這次發作的時後，我的意識非常清楚。

□ Sometimes, the left side of my body feels really weak.
有時候我會覺得身體左側軟弱無力。

□ I had a CT scan[2] and an EEG,[3] but they can't seem to find the problem.
我做過電腦斷層掃描和腦波檢查，但是似乎找不出問題所在。

□ I used to take medication for it, but after three years of no seizures, my doctor thought I could stop.
我以前吃有吃抑制的藥物，但是因為之後三年都沒發作，我的醫生認為我可以停。

□ Is it possible that something else is causing my seizures?
我的發作有沒有可能是其他因素所引起的？

Word List ▸▸▸

1 conscious [ˋkɑnʃəs] *adj.* 有知覺的；有意識的
2 CT scan = computerized axial tomography scan [kəmˋpjutɚˏraɪzd ˋæksɪəl təˋmɑgrəfɪ ˏskæn] 電腦斷層掃描
3 EEG = electroencephalogram [ɪˏlɛtroɛnˋsɛfələˏgræm] 腦電波；腦動電流圖

醫病診療 *900* 句典 **129**

108 噎住 I ──醫護人員的指示

☐ See if he can speak or cough first.

先看他是否能開口說話或咳嗽。

☐ Try to see if something is stuck[1] in her airway.[2]

看看是不是有異物卡在她的呼吸道裡。

☐ If you can see what's blocking the airway, reach in and try to sweep[3] it away. Be careful not to push it deeper into the airway.

如果你可以看到是什麼東西卡在呼吸道裡，手伸進去把它挪到一邊。小心不要把東西往裡面推。

☐ There's no time to get her to the hospital. Help her right now.

沒時間送她到醫院了，現在就幫她。

☐ Perform the Heimlich maneuver[4] until the blockage[5] is dislodged.[6]

實行哈姆立克急救法，直到移除堵塞物為止。

☐ We'll need to take an X-ray to make sure nothing else is stuck in the airway.

我們需要照 X 光以確認沒有其他東西卡在呼吸道裡。

Word List ▸ ▸ ▸

1 stuck [stʌk] *adj.* 卡住的

2 airway [ˈɛr,we] *n.* 呼吸道

3 sweep [swip] *v.* 掃除；掃去

4 Heimlich maneuver [ˈhaɪmlɪk məˌnuvɚ]
n. 漢默李奇急救法（使堵住喉嚨的異物吐出的急救措施）

5 block [ˈblɑk] *v.* 封鎖；堵塞

6 dislodged [dɪsˈlɑdʒ] *v.* 把……移去

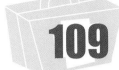

109 噎住 II ── 你可以這麼說

□ He's not breathing! Help! He's turning blue![1]
他沒呼吸了！救命！他臉色發青了。

□ Does anyone know the Heimlich maneuver?
有沒有人會做哈姆立克急救法？

□ She's unconscious. Does anyone know CPR?
她沒有意識了。有沒有人會做心肺復甦術？

□ He was talking and eating at the same time.
他邊說話邊吃東西。

□ I think my daughter swallowed[2] part of a toy or something.
我想我的女兒把玩具零件還是什麼的吞下去了。

□ He vomited in his sleep.
他睡覺時嘔吐。

10

意外和緊急事件

Word List ▶▶▶

1 turn blue 臉色發青

2 swallow [`swɑlo] v. 吞下；嚥下

110 呼吸障礙 I ——描述症狀

☐ I can't breathe!

我不能呼吸！

☐ I was just walking, and suddenly I got completely winded.¹

我只不過在走著，突然之間卻完全喘不過氣來。

☐ I couldn't get any air into my lungs.

我沒辦法呼吸。

☐ I think I'm having an asthma attack.²

我想我的氣喘要發作了。

☐ If I do anything strenuous³ I start gasping⁴ for air.

如果我做點費力的事情就會氣喘如牛。

☐ When I start to wheeze,⁵ I panic,⁶ and it makes it worse.

我只要一氣喘就會驚慌，然後情形就更糟。

Word List ▶▶▶

1 winded [ˋwɪndɪd] *adj.* 喘氣的；喘不過氣來的
2 asthma attack [ˋæzmə ə.tæk] *n.* 氣喘發作
3 strenuous [ˋstrɛnjuəs] *adj.* 費力的

4 gasp [gæsp] *v.* 喘氣
5 wheeze [hwiz] *v.* 發出氣喘的聲音
6 panic [ˋpænɪk] *v.* 恐慌；驚慌

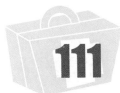

111 呼吸障礙 II ——醫護人員的回應

☐ Do you ever lose consciousness when you're having trouble breathing?

你呼吸困難時會不會失去意識？

☐ You might suffer from acute[1] anxiety[2] attacks.

你可能得了急性焦慮症。

☐ Your body went into shock.[3] Are you allergic to anything?

你的身體產生休克。你是不是對什麼東西過敏？

☐ Are you taking any drugs?[4]

你是不是正在服用什麼藥物？

☐ Have you suffered any injuries to the chest[5] area lately?

你最近胸部有沒有受過什麼傷？

☐ How many cigarettes do you smoke each day?

你一天抽幾根菸？

Word List ▶▶▶

1 acute [ə`kjut] *adj.* 急性的

2 anxiety [æŋ`zaɪətɪ] *n.* 焦慮；掛念

3 shock [ʃɑk] *n.* 休克

4 drug [drʌg] *n.* 藥品；藥材

5 chest [tʃɛst] *n.* 胸；胸膛

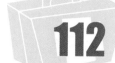
112 溺水 I ──醫護人員可能這麼說

☐ How long was he under the water for?
他在水面下待了多久？

☐ Did he regain[1] consciousness after you pulled him out?
你把他拉出來之後他有沒有恢復意識？

☐ Oxygen[2] was cut off to her brain.[3] We'll have to monitor[4] her condition.
她腦部缺氧。我們必須監控她的狀況。

☐ He had a lot of water in his lungs.
他的肺部積了很多水。

☐ She's being treated for hypothermia.[5]
她因體溫過低正在接受治療。

☐ It's too early to know, but your friend may have suffered some brain damage.[6]
現在還不能確定，但是你的朋友腦部可能受了損害。

Word List ▶▶▶

1 regain [rɪ`gen] v. 恢復
2 oxygen [`ɑksədʒən] n. 氧（氣）
3 brain [bren] n. 腦
4 monitor [`mɑnətə] n. 監視器

5 hypothermia [ˌhaɪpə`θɜmɪə] n. 體溫過低（症）
6 damage [`dæmɪdʒ] n. 損害

113 溺水 II ── 你可以這麼說

□ He was probably in the water for only 2 minutes.

他可能在水裡只待了兩分鐘。

□ When we pulled her out, she started coughing up[1] water.

我們把她拉出來的時候,她就開始咳水出來。

□ It looked like he swallowed a lot of water.

看起來他似乎吃進了很多水。

□ The lifeguard gave her mouth-to-mouth[2] resuscitation.

救生人員對她進行口對口人工呼吸。

□ Will this incident[3] affect him in any other way?

發生這個事會不會對他造成任何影響?

□ Is there any chance of a full recovery?[4]

有沒有可能完全復原?

10

意外和緊急事件

Word List ▶▶▶

1 cough up 咳出

2 mouth-to-mouth resuscitation
[ˋmauθtəˋmauθ rɪˌsʌsəˋteʃən] n. 口對口人
工呼吸

3 incident [ˋɪnsədənt] n. 事件

4 full recovery 完全的復原

114 中風 I ——醫護人員可能這麼說

☐ You've suffered a small stroke,[1] but you're going to be fine.
你有輕微的中風，但是不會有事。

☐ Try to raise both arms and keep them raised.
試著把兩隻手臂舉起來，然後保持那個姿勢。

☐ A blood clot[2] in his brain caused the stroke.
他腦中的一個血塊引起了中風。

☐ A blood vessel[3] in her brain is leaking.[4] That's what caused the mild stroke.
她的一根腦血管溢血，這是造成輕微中風的原因。

☐ I'm going to inject you with a clot-busting drug.[5]
我要為你注射抗凝血藥劑。

☐ We'll need to perform surgery to improve blood flow[6] to the brain.
我們需要進行手術以改善流向腦部的血流。

Word List ▶▶▶

1 stroke [strok] *n.* 中風
2 clot [klɑt] *n.* （血等的）凝塊
3 vessel [ˈvɛsl] *n.* 血管
4 leak [lik] *v.* 漏

5 clot-busting drug [ˈklɑt͵bʌstɪŋ`drʌg] *n.* 抗凝血藥劑
6 blood flow [ˈblʌd͵flo] *n.* 血的流動

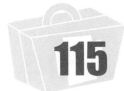

115 中風 II ── 你可以這麼說

☐ The left side of my body suddenly felt numb.[1]
我身體的左半邊突然感覺麻木。

☐ She seems to have trouble talking. Her speech is slurred.[2]
她說話好像有困難，口齒不清。

☐ Sometimes my vision is blurred, or I see double.
我有時候會視線模糊，有時候會看見雙重影像。

☐ Has the stroke caused any permanent[3] damage?
中風有沒有造成任何永久性的傷害？

☐ Will he regain full control[4] of his facial[5] muscles?
他的顏面神經會完全回復自主嗎？

☐ Besides physical therapy,[6] is there any other treatment?
除了物理治療外，還有其他療法嗎？

10

意外和緊急事件

Word List ▶▶▶

1 numb [nʌm] *adj.* 失去感覺的；麻木的

2 slurred [slɜd] *adj.* 發音含糊的

3 permanent [ˈpɜmənənt] *adj.* 永恆的；永久的

4 regain full control 恢復完全自主

5 facial [ˈfeʃəl] *adj.* 臉的；面部的

6 physical therapy [ˈfɪzɪkl̩ ˈθɛrəpɪ] 物理療法

116 心臟病 I ——醫護人員可能這麼說

☐ Are you feeling any discomfort in other areas of your body?
你身體的其他部位有沒有覺得不舒服？

☐ Are you on any heart medication?
你有沒有在服用任何心臟疾病的藥？

☐ Do you have a history of heart disease[1] in your family?
你的家族有沒有心臟病史？

☐ You'll need an angioplasty[2] to open up your arteries.[3]
你需要進行血管修復術把你的動脈打通。

☐ It looks like you had an episode of angina.[4]
看起來你是出現了心絞痛。

☐ The heart attack severely damaged your heart.
你心臟病發作嚴重損害了你的心臟。

Word List ▶▶▶

1 history of a disease 病史（通常指家族中某種常發生的疾病）

2 angioplasty [ˈændʒɪə͵plæstɪ] n. 血管修復術

3 artery [ˈɑrtərɪ] n. 動脈

4 angina [ænˈdʒaɪnə] n. 心絞痛；咽喉痛；咽峽炎

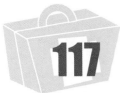

117 心臟病 II —— 你可以這麼說

☐ My left arm tingles.[1]
我的左手臂有刺痛感。

☐ There's a stabbing[2] pain in my chest.
我胸部的疼痛有如刀刺。

☐ He just clutched his chest[3] and collapsed.[4]
他就只緊抓著胸部，接著就昏倒了。

☐ I had a mild heart attack five years ago.
我五年前心臟病曾輕微發作過。

☐ I've been taking aspirin for my heart condition.
我一直在服用阿斯匹靈控制我心臟的狀況。

☐ Am I at risk for[5] another heart attack?
我是不是有心臟病復發的危險？

Word List ▶ ▶ ▶

1 tingle [ˈtɪŋgl] *n.* 刺痛
2 stabbing [ˈstæbɪŋ] *adj.* 如刀刺的
3 chest [tʃɛst] *n.* 胸膛

4 collapse [kəˈlæps] *v.* 倒塌；倒下
5 at risk for 有……的危險

Part 11

找專科醫師

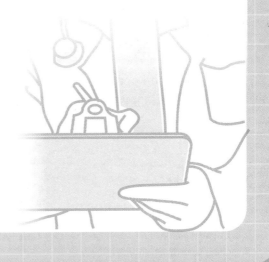

118 上婦產科 I ——描述症狀

☐ I haven't had a period[1] in two months.
　我的月經已經兩個月沒來了。

☐ I get really bad cramps[2] during my period.
　我月經來的時候腹部絞痛得很厲害。

☐ It's really itchy[3] down there.
　下面那邊好癢。

☐ My period came two weeks ago, but I still have some spotting.[4]
　我的月經是兩個禮拜以前來的，但是到現在我仍然還有一些些血。

☐ I think I have a yeast infection.[5]
　我想我感染了陰道炎。

☐ It burns when I pee.[6]
　我小解的時候有灼熱感。

Word List ▶▶▶

1 period [ˈpɪrɪəd] *n.* 月經
2 cramp [kræmp] *n.* 抽筋；痙攣
3 itchy [ˈɪtʃɪ] *adj.* 癢的
4 spotting [ˈspɑtɪŋ] *n.* （雨、血等）小點

5 yeast infection [ˈjist ɪn.fɛkʃən] *n.* 黴菌陰道感染
6 pee [pi] *v.* 撒尿；小便

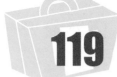
119 上婦產科 II——醫護人員可以這樣說

☐ Have you had any unusual[1] discharge?[2]

妳有沒有不尋常的分泌物？

☐ How long do your periods usually last for?

妳的月經通常持續多久？

☐ Are you on birth control?[3]

妳是不是在避孕？

☐ Have you ever been pregnant?[4]

妳有沒有懷過孕？

☐ After you put on this gown, lie down in the examination chair and place your feet in the stirrups.[5] The doctor will be with your shortly.

妳穿上這件長袍之後，躺在診察椅上，把腳放在腳鐙裡。醫生很快就來。

☐ Have you noticed any unusual odors?[6]

妳有沒有注意到任何異常的味道？

11

找專科醫師

Word List ▶▶▶

1 unusual [ʌnˋjuɛʊəl] *adj.* 異常的

2 discharge [dɪsˋtʃɑrdʒ] *n.* 排出或流出的液體或氣體

3 birth control 生育控制；避孕

4 pregnant [ˋprɛgnənt] *adj.* 懷孕的

5 stirrup [ˋstɜəp] *n.* 鐙具

6 odor [ˋodə] *n.* 氣味

120 看牙醫 I——描述症狀

☐ I have a really bad toothache.¹
我的牙真的痛得很厲害。

☐ I fell down and chipped² my front tooth.
我跌倒，門牙撞缺了一角。

☐ I lost a filling.³
我牙齒的填充物掉了。

☐ My teeth are really sensitive⁴ to cold.
我的牙齒對冷非常敏感。

☐ My gums⁵ seem a little swollen.
我的牙齦好像有一點腫。

☐ Do you do teeth whitening?⁶
你們有沒有做牙齒漂白？

Word List ▶▶▶

1 toothache [ˈtuθ͵ek] *n.* 牙痛
2 chip [tʃɪp] *v.* 削去；弄缺
3 filling [ˈfɪlɪŋ] *n.* 填補蛀牙的填充物
4 sensitive [ˈsɛnsətɪv] *adj.* 敏感的；神經過敏的

5 gum [gʌm] *n.* 牙齦；牙床（常用複數）
6 teeth whitening [ˈtiθ ˈhwaɪtṇɪŋ] *n.* 牙齒漂白

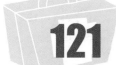

121 看牙醫 II ——醫護人員可以這樣說

☐ Do you get your teeth cleaned regularly?

你有沒有定期清潔牙齒？

☐ Would you prefer a metal[1] or a white filling?[2]

你補牙要選擇用金屬還是合成樹脂？

☐ When did you get this crown[3] put in?

你這個齒冠是什麼時候裝的？

☐ Do you floss?[4]

你有沒有使用牙線？

☐ It looks like you have two new cavities.[5]

看起來你有兩顆新的蛀牙。

☐ Your tooth is infected. I'll have to do a root canal.[6]

你的牙齒發炎了。我得進行根管治療。

Word List ▶ ▶ ▶

1 metal [ˈmɛtl] *n.* 金屬

2 white filling [ˈhwaɪt ˌfɪlɪŋ] *n.* 合成樹脂填牙

3 floss [flɔs] *v.* 用牙線潔牙

4 cavity [ˈkævətɪ] *n.* 蛀洞

5 root canal [ˈrut kəˌnæl] *n.* 牙齒的根管治療

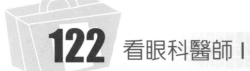
☐ My eyes have been really red and watery lately.

最近我的眼睛很紅又會流眼油。

☐ My eyes are really sensitive to light.

我的眼睛對光線非常敏感。

☐ I think I might have night blindness.[1]

我想我可能得了夜盲症。

☐ It feels like there's something in my eye.

我眼睛感覺好像有東西跑進去。

☐ I keep seeing a blurry[2] shape[3] out of my left eye.

我的左眼一直看到一個模糊的影子。

☐ I see haloes[4] around lights.

我看光的時都覺得有光暈。

Word List ▶ ▶ ▶

1 night blindness [ˋnaɪt͵blaɪndnɪs] *n.* 夜盲   3 shape [ʃep] *n.* 形象；輪廓

2 blurry [ˋblɜɪ] *adj.* 模糊的   4 halo [ˋhelo] *n.* 光環；光澤

123 看眼科醫師 II —— 醫師的回應

☐ Is the pain in or around the eye?

痛是在眼睛裡面，還是在眼睛周圍？

☐ Any problem with your peripheral[1] vision?[2]

你的周邊視野有沒有問題？

☐ We'll see how your pupils[3] respond to[4] light.

我們要看看你的瞳孔對光有何反應。

☐ I'm going to use some eyedrops to dilate[5] your pupils.

我要點一些眼藥水讓你的瞳孔擴張。

☐ You'll need surgery to remove the cataract.[6]

你需要動手術移除白內障。

☐ Does it hurt when you squint?[7]

你瞇眼睛的時候會不會痛？

11

找專科醫師

Word List ▶ ▶ ▶

1 peripheral [pəˋrɪfərəl] *adj.* 周圍的（神經）
  末梢的

2 vision [ˋvɪʒən] *n.* 視力；視覺；視野

3 pupil [ˋpjupl] *n.* 瞳孔

4 respond to 對……有反應

5 dilate [daɪˋlet] *v.* 擴大

6 cataract [ˋkætəˌrækt] *n.* 白內障

7 squint [skwɪnt] *v.* 瞇著眼睛看；斜視

Part 12

字彙與圖示

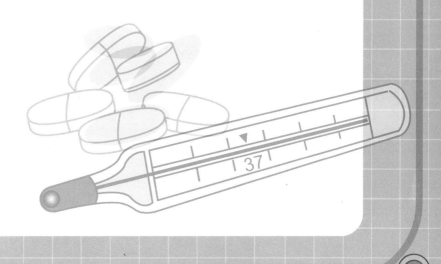

124 頭部相關字彙

1. head [hɛd] *n.* 頭
2. forehead [ˈfɔr͵hɛd] *n.* 額頭
3. ear [ɪr] *n.* 耳
    i. earlobe [ˈɪr͵lob] *n.* 耳垂
4. eye [aɪ] *n.* 眼睛
    i. eyebrow [ˈaɪ͵braʊ] *n.* 眉毛
    ii. eyelash [ˈaɪ͵læʃ] *n.* 睫毛
    iii. eyelid [ˈaɪ͵lɪd] *n.* 眼皮
    iv. iris [ˈaɪrɪs] *n.*（眼球的）虹膜
    v. pupil [ˈpjupl̩] *n.* 瞳孔
    vi. the white of one's eye 眼白
5. nose [noz] *n.* 鼻子
    i. bridge of the nose 鼻樑
    ii. nostril [ˈnɑstrɪl] *n.* 鼻孔
6. mouth [maʊθ] *n.* 嘴
    i. lip [lɪp] *n.* 嘴唇
    ii. tongue [tʌŋ] *n.* 舌頭
    iii. teeth [tiθ] *n.* 牙齒（tooth [tuθ] 之複數形）

iv. jaw [dʒɔ] *n.* 顎
v. chin [tʃɪn] *n.* 下巴
7. cheek [tʃik] *n.* 臉頰
8. neck [nɛk] *n.* 脖子
    i. nape [nep] (of one's neck) *n.* 頸背
    ii. Adam's apple 喉結

125 頭部圖示

4

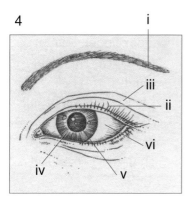

i
iii
ii
vi
iv
v

6

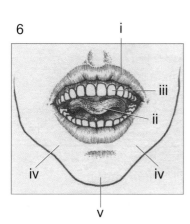

i
iii
ii
iv
iv
v

1

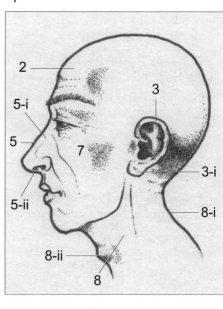

2
3
5-i
5
7
5-ii
3-i
8-i
8-ii
8

12

字彙與圖示

126 身體相關字彙

1. torso [ˈtɔrso] *n.* 軀幹
   i. shoulder [ˈʃoldə] *n.* 肩膀
   ii. back [bæk] *n.* 背
   iii. chest [tʃɛst] *n.* 胸
   iv. breast [brɛst] *n.* 乳房
   v. waist [west] *n.* 腰
   vi. belly button [ˈbɛlɪˌbʌtn̩] *n.* 肚臍
   vii. hip [hɪp] *n.* 臀部
   viii. buttocks [ˈbʌtəks] *n.* 屁股
   ix. penis [ˈpinɪs] *n.* 陰莖
   x. vagina [vəˈdʒaɪnə] *n.* 陰道
2. arm [ɑrm] *n.* 手臂
   i. upper arm [ˈʌpəˈɑrm] *n.* 上臂
   ii. elbow [ˈɛlbo] *n.* 肘
   iii. forearm [ˈforˌɑrm] *n.* 前臂
   iv. wrist [rɪst] *n.* 腕
3. hand [hænd] *n.* 手
   i. back of the hand 手背
   ii. palm [pɑm] (of the hand) *n.* 手心；手掌
   iii. finger [ˈfɪŋgə] (pinky, ring finger, middle finger, index finger, thumb) ([ˈpɪŋkɪ] / [ˈrɪŋˌfɪŋgə] / [ˈmɪdl̩ˈfɪŋgə] / [ˈɪndɛksˌfɪŋgə] / [θʌm]) *n.* 手指（小指、無名指、中指、食指、拇指）
   iv. fingernail [ˈfɪŋgəˌnel] *n.* 指甲
4. leg [lɛg] *n.* 腿
   i. thigh [θaɪ] *n.* 大腿
   ii. calf [kæf] *n.* 小腿
5. knee [ni] *n.* 膝蓋
6. ankle [ˈæŋkl̩] *n.* 腳踝
7. foot [fʊt] *n.* 腳
   i. ball of the foot 大腳指底部的肉球
   ii. heel [hil] *n.* 腳後跟
   iii. arch [ɑrtʃ] *n.*
   iv. toe [to] *n.* 腳指
   v. toenail [ˈtoˌnel] *n.* 腳指甲

127 身體圖示

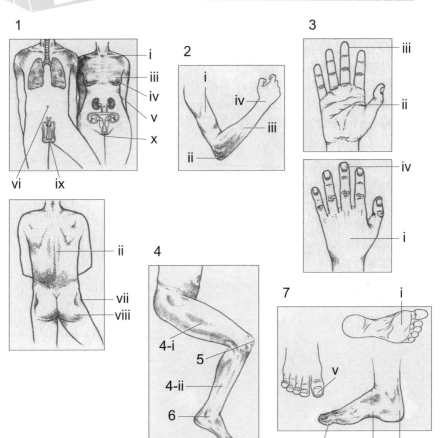

128 內部器官相關字彙

1. heart [hɑrt] *n.* 心
2. lung [lʌŋ] *n.* 肺
3. stomach [ˋstʌmək] *n.* 胃
4. gallbladder [ˋgɔl͵blædɚ] *n.* 膽囊
5. small intestine [ˋsmɔl͵ ɪnˋtɛstɪn] *n.* 小腸
6. large intestine [lɑrdʒ͵ ɪnˋtɛstɪn] *n.* 大腸
7. colon [ˋkolən] *n.* 結腸
8. liver [ˋlɪvɚ] *n.* 肝
9. kidney [ˋkɪdnɪ] *n.* 腎
10. pancreas [ˋpæŋkrɪəs] *n.* 胰臟
11. spleen [splin] *n.* 脾臟
12. appendix [əˋpɛndɪks] *n.* 盲腸；闌尾
13. diaphragm [ˋdaɪə͵fræm] *n.* 橫隔膜

129 内部器官圖示

1
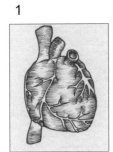

2
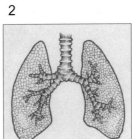

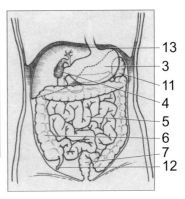

13
3
11
4
5
6
7
12

8
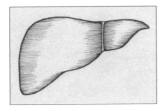

9
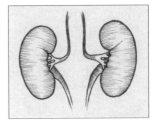

10
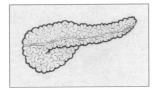

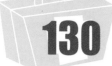
130 骨骼相關字彙

1. skull [skʌl] *n.* 頭蓋骨
2. torso [tɔrso] *n.* 軀幹
   i. spine [spaɪn] / back-bone [ˋbæk͵bon] *n.* 脊椎
   ii. vertebrae [ˋvɜtəbri] *n.* 脊椎骨（verterbra [ˋvɜtəbrə] 之複數形）
   iii. collarbone [ˋkɑlɚ͵bon] / clavicle [ˋklævəkl̩] *n.* 鎖骨
   iv. shoulder blade [ˋʃoldɚ͵bled] / scapula [ˋskæpjələ] *n.* 肩胛骨
   v. breastbone [ˋbrɛst͵bon] / sternum [ˋstɜnəm] *n.* 胸骨
   vi. rib [rɪb] *n.* 肋骨
   vii. rib cage [ˋrɪb͵kedʒ] *n.* 胸腔
   viii. pelvis [ˋpɛlvɪs] *n.* 骨盆
   ix. tailbone [ˋtel͵bon] / coccyx [ˋkɑksɪks] *n.* 尾椎骨

3. arms and hands 手臂和手
   i. humerus [ˋhjumərəs] *n.* 肱骨
   ii. ulna [ˋʌlnə] *n.* 尺骨
   iii. radius [ˋredɪəs] *n.* 橈骨
   iv. carpal bone [ˋkɑrpl̩͵bon] *n.* 腕骨
   v. metacarpal bone [͵mɛtəˋkɑrpl̩͵bon] *n.* 掌骨
   vi. phalange [ˋfæləndʒ] *n.* （手）指骨

4. legs 腿
   i. femur [ˋfimə] *n.* 股骨
   ii. tibia [ˋtɪbɪə] *n.* 脛骨
   iii. fibula [ˋfɪbjələ] *n.* 腓骨
   iv. tarsal bone [ˋtɑrsl̩͵bon] *n.* 跗骨
   v. metatarsal bone [͵mɛtəˋtɑrsəl͵bon] *n.* 蹠骨
   vi. phalanges [ˋfæləndʒ] *n.* （腳）指骨

131 骨骼圖示

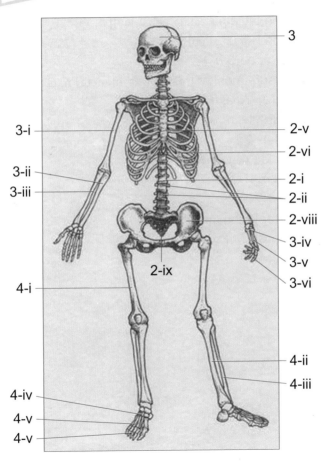

3

3-i

3-ii

3-iii

2-v

2-vi

2-i

2-ii

2-viii

3-iv

3-v

3-vi

2-ix

4-i

4-ii

4-iii

4-iv

4-v

4-v

132 醫生診療室內相關字彙

1. examination table [ɪɡˌzæməˋneʃənˌtebl̩] *n.* 診療台
2. stethoscope [ˋstɛθəˌskop] *n.* 聽診器
3. eye chart [ˋaɪˌtʃɑrt] *n.* 視力檢查表
4. blood pressure monitor [ˋblʌdˌprɛʃəˌmɑnətə] *n.* 血壓計
5. ear scope [ˋɪrˌskop] *n.* 內視潔耳器
6. syringe [ˋsɪrɪndʒ] *n.* 注射器
7. nurse [nɜs] *n.* 護士
8. paper towels [ˋpepəˌtauəl] *n.* 紙巾
9. scale [skel] *n.* 秤
10. sink [sɪŋk] *n.* 水槽
11. thermometer [θəˋmɑmətə] *n.* 溫度計
12. tongue depressor [ˋtʌŋdɪˌprɛsə] *n.* 壓舌板

醫生診療室內圖示

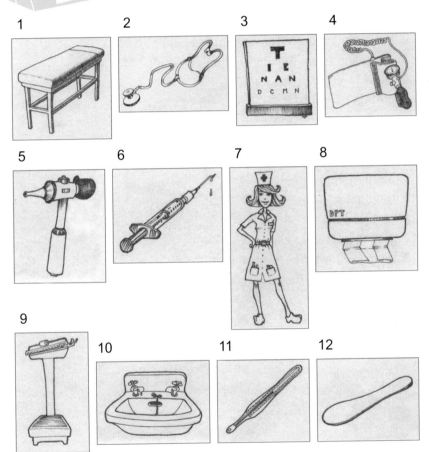

1

2

3

4

5

6

7

8

9

10

11

12

12

字彙與圖示

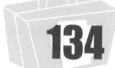

134 醫院內設備相關字彙與圖示

1. receptionist [rɪ`sɛpʃənɪst] *n.* 接待員
2. examination room [ɪg͵zæmə`neʃən rum] *n.* 診療室
3. operating room [`ɑpə͵retɪŋ ͵rum] *n.* 手術房
4. ward [wɔrd] *n.* 病房
5. curtain [`kɜtn̩] *n.* 帷幔
6. gurney [`gɜnɪ] *n.* 輪床
7. wheelchair [`hwil͵tʃɛr] *n.* 輪椅
8. patient's chart [`peʃənts`tʃɑrt] *n.* 病歷表
9. bandages [`bændɪdʒ] *n.* 繃帶
10. tray [tre] *n.* 托盤
11. cart [kɑrt] *n.* 置物櫃推車
12. gloves [glʌvz] *n.* 手套（複數）
13. hospital gown [`hɑspɪtl͵gaʊn] *n.* 醫生袍
14. scrubs [skrʌbz] *n.* 開刀服（複數形，包括上身下身）
15. mask [mæsk] *n.* 口罩
16. monitor [`mɑnətɚ] *n.* 監視器
17. gift shop [`gɪft͵ʃɑp] *n.* 禮品店

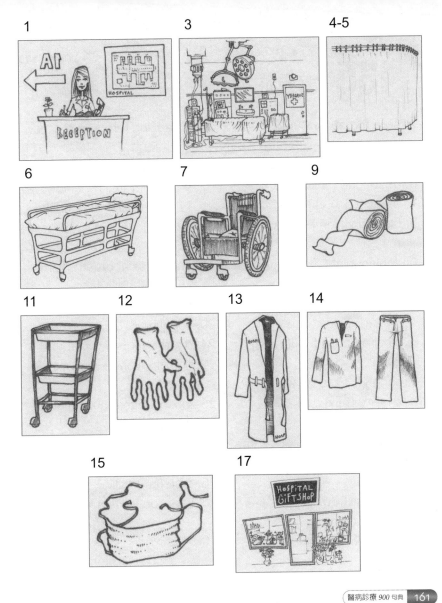

1

3

4-5

6

7

9

11

12

13

14

15

17

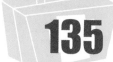

1. sore throat [ˋsorˋθrot] n. 喉嚨痛
2. fever [ˋfivɚ] n. 發燒
3. headache [ˋhɛdˏek] n. 頭痛
4. earache [ˋɪrˏek] n. 耳痛
5. blurred vision [ˋblɝdˋvɪʒən] n. 眼花
6. aching joint [ˋekɪŋˋdʒɔɪnt] n. 關節疼痛
7. runny nose [ˋrʌnɪˋnoz] n. 流鼻水
8. blocked nose [ˋblɑktˋnoz] n. 鼻塞
9. cough [kɔf] n./v. 咳嗽
10. sneeze [sniz] n./v. 打噴嚏
11. phlegm [flɛm] n. 痰
12. shiver [ˋʃɪvɚ] n./v. 顫抖
13. cold sweat [ˋkoldˋswɛt] n. 冷汗
14. dizziness [ˋdɪzɪnɪs] n. 頭昏眼花
15. muscle cramp [ˋmʌsļˏkræmp] n. 肌肉抽筋
16. wheezing [ˋhwizɪŋ] n. 氣喘所發出的聲音
17. abdominal [æbˋdɑmənļ] / shoulder [ˋʃoldɚ] / elbow [ˋɛlbo] / neck [nɛk] / back / chest [tʃɛst] pain n. 肚子／肩膀／手肘／脖子／背部／胸部痛
18. shortness of breath [ˋʃɔrtnɪs əv ˋbrɛθ] n. 呼吸困難
19. nausea [ˋnɔʃɪə] n. 噁心；作嘔
20. vomiting [ˋvɑmɪtɪŋ] n. 嘔吐
21. diarrhea [ˏdaɪəˋriə] n. 腹瀉
22. constipation [ˏkɑnstəˋpeʃən] n. 便秘
23. incontinence [ɪnˋkɑntənəns] n. 大小便失禁
24. swelling [ˋswɛlɪŋ] n. 腫瘤；疙瘩；瘤；腫起部分
25. rash [ræʃ] n. 疹子
26. infection [ɪnˋfɛkʃən] n. 感染

136 常見疾病或健康問題

1. cold [kold] *n.* 感冒
2. cold sore [`kold, sor] *n.*（傷風、發熱時出現的）唇皰疹；嘴邊皰疹
3. flu [flu] *n.* 流行性感冒
4. pneumonia [nju`monjə] *n.* 肺炎
5. asthma [`æzmə] *n.* 氣喘（病）；哮喘
6. whooping cough [`hupɪŋ, kɔf] *n.* 百日咳
7. tonsillitis [, tɑnsḷ`aɪtɪs] *n.* 扁桃腺炎
8. chicken pox [`tʃɪkən, pɑks] *n.* 水痘
9. botulin [`bɑtʃəlɪn] *n.* 肉毒桿菌
10. cholera [`kɑlərə] *n.* 霍亂
11. diphtheria [dɪf`θɪrɪə] *n.* 白喉
12. E. coli [`ɪ`kolaɪ] *n.* 大腸桿菌
13. malaria [mə`lɛrɪə] *n.* 瘧疾
14. measles [`mizḷz] *n.* 麻疹
15. meningitis [, mɛnɪn`dʒaɪtɪs] *n.* 腦膜炎
16. rabies [`rebiz] *n.* 狂犬病
17. rubella [ru`bɛlə] *n.* 德國麻疹
18. tetanus [`tɛtənəs] *n.* 破傷風
19. tuberculosis [tju, bɝkjə`losɪs] *n.* 肺結核
20. typhoid [`taɪfɔɪd] *n.* 傷寒
21. dysentery [`dɪsṇ, tɛrɪ] *n.* 痢疾
22. salmonella [, sælmə`nɛlə] *n.* 沙門氏菌
23. strep throat [`strɛp, θrot] *n.* 鏈球菌性喉炎
24. genital warts [`dʒɛnətḷ`wɔrts] *n.* 生殖器疣；性器疣（俗稱椰菜花）
25. gonorrhea [, gɑnə`riə] *n.* 淋病
26. herpes [`hɝpiz] *n.* 皰疹
27. syphilis [`sɪflɪs] *n.* 梅毒
28. AIDS [edz] *n.* 愛滋病；後天性免疫不全症候群（= acquired immunodeficiency syndrome [ə`kwaɪrd ɪ, mjənodɪ`fɪʃənsɪ , sɪndrom]）

29. yeast infection
['jistɪn, fɛkʃən] *n.* 黴菌陰道感染

30. bladder infection ['blædə
ɪn, fɛkʃən] *n.* 膀胱感染

31. appendicitis [ə, pɛndə`saɪtɪs]
n. 闌尾炎；盲腸炎

32. arthritis [ɑr`θraɪtɪs] *n.* 關節炎

33. athlete's foot ['æθlits`fut] *n.*
香港腳

34. encephalitis [, ɛnsɛfə`laɪtɪs]
n. 腦炎

35. mumps [mʌmps] *n.* 耳下腺
炎；腮腺炎

36. cancer ['kænsə] *n.* 癌症

37. cardiac arrest ['kɑrdɪ, æk
ə`rɛst] *n.* 心搏停止；心臟停跳

38. hepatitis [, hɛpə`taɪtɪs] A / B /
C / E *n.* （A / B / C / E）型肝
炎

39. leukemia [lu`kimɪə] *n.* 白血病
（俗稱血癌）

40. anemia [ə`nimɪə] *n.* 貧血

41. mono ['mɑno] *n.* 單核白血球
增多症（= mononucleosis
[, mɑno, nuklɪ`osɪs]）

42. lyme disease ['laɪm, dɪziz] 萊
姆症（又稱萊姆關節炎，由扁蝨
傳染，症狀有紅斑、頭疼、發燒
等等）

43. wart [wɔrt] *n.* 疣

44. migraine ['maɪgren] *n.* 偏頭痛

45. irritable bowel syndrome
['ɪrətəbl̩`bauəl, sɪndrom] *n.* 大
腸急躁症

46. myopia [maɪ`opɪə] *n.* 近視

47. hypermetropia
[, haɪpəmə`tropɪə] *n.* 遠視

48. astigmatism [ə`stɪgmə, tɪzəm]
n. 散光

49. chronic fatigue syndrome
['krɑnɪkfə`tig, sɪndrom] *n.* 慢
性疲勞症

50. alzheimer's ['alts, haɪməz]
（disease） *n.* 老年癡呆症

Part **13**

參考資訊

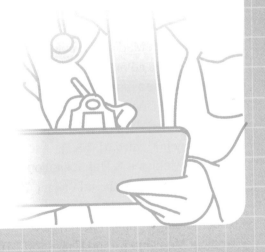

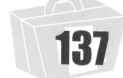

137 醫院部門

醫學名詞通常又長又複雜。以下列出醫院部門名稱，有助於你尋求協助。

- Anesthesiology [ˌænəsˌθizɪˈɑlədʒɪ] 麻醉科
- Cardiothoracic Surgery [ˌkɑrdɪoθoˈræsɪkˈsɜdʒərɪ] 胸腔外科手術
- Dermatology [ˌdɜməˈtɑlədʒɪ] 皮膚科
- Allergy & Immunology [ˈælədʒɪændˌɪmjəˈnɑlədʒɪ] 過敏免疫科
- Cardiovascular Disease [ˌkɑrdɪoˈvæskjulədɪˈziz] 心臟血管疾病科
- Critical Care Medicine [ˈkrɪtɪkḷˈkɛrˌmɛdəsṇ] 重症醫學科
- Emergency Services [ɪˈmɜdʒənsɪˌsɜvɪs] 急診醫學科
- Endocrinology [ˌɛndokrɪˈnɑlədʒɪ] / Metabolism [məˈtæbḷˌɪzəm] 內分泌／新陳代謝科
- Gastroenterology [ˌgæstroˌɛntəˈrɑlədʒɪ] 腸胃科
- Hematology & Medical Oncology [ˌhiməˈtɑlədʒɪændˈmɛdɪkḷˌɑŋˈkɑlədʒɪ] 腫瘤血液科
- Infectious Diseases [ɪnˈfɛkʃəs dɪˈzizɪz] 傳染病科
- Internal Medicine [ɪnˈtɜnḷˈmɛdəsṇ] / Primary Care [ˈpraɪˌmərɪˈkɛr] 內科／基層護理
- Neurology [njuˈrɑlədʒɪ] 神經科
- Physical Medicine & Rehabilitation [ˈfɪzɪkḷˈmɛdəsṇændˌrihəˌbɪləˈteʃən] 復健醫學科
- Pulmonary Medicine [ˈpʌlməˌnɛrɪˈmɛdəsṇ] 肺腔醫學科
- Rheumatology [ˌruməˈtɑlədʒɪ] 風濕科
- Tropical Medicine [ˈtrɑpɪkḷˈmɛdəsṇ] / Tropical Disease

［ˈtrɑpɪkḷ dɪˋziz] 熱帶醫學／熱帶疾病科

- Obstetrics & Gynecology [əbˋstɛtrɪksænd͵gaɪnəˋkɑlədʒɪ] 婦產科
- Ophthalmology [͵ɑfθælˋmɑlədʒɪ] 眼科
- Orthopedic Surgery [͵ɔrθəˋpidɪk ˋsɜdʒərɪ] 整形外科
- Otolaryngology [͵otə͵ærɪŋˋgɑlədʒɪ] / Head & Neck Surgery
  [ˋhɛdændˋnɛk͵sɜdʒərɪ] 耳鼻喉科／頭頸外科
- Dentistry & Oral Surgery [ˋdɛntɪstrɪændˋorəlˋsɜdʒərɪ] 牙科與口腔外科
- Pathology [pəˋθɑlədʒɪ] 病理學
- Pediatrics [͵pidɪˋætrɪks] 小兒科
- Psychiatry [saɪˋkaɪətrɪ] 精神科
- Radiology [͵redɪˋɑlədʒɪ] 放射科
- Surgery [ˋsɜdʒərɪ] 外科
- General Surgery [ˋdʒɛnərəl ˋsɜdʒərɪ] 一般外科
- Neurosurgery [͵njuroˋsɜdʒərɪ] 神經外科
- Plastic & Reconstructive Surgery
  [ˋplæstɪkænd͵rikənˋstrʌktɪvˋsɜdʒərɪ] 重健整形外科
- Urology [juˋrɑlədʒɪ] 泌尿科
- Vascular Surgery [ˋvæskjələ ˋsɜdʒərɪ] 血管外科

138 看診時尋求其他協助

善用下列建議，以確保自己能掌握所有就醫情況。

1) 詢問醫院是否提供翻譯服務。

☞ For example: "My English isn't very good. Do you have a translator?"

例如：「我的英文不太好，你們有翻譯人員嗎？」

2) 確定醫院或醫師看過你的病歷文件，確定他們知道你是否正在服用任何藥物，或者對什麼過敏。

☞ For example: "I'm allergic to aspirin."、"I'm taking Percocet for my back pain"

例如：「我對阿斯匹靈過敏。」、「我正在服用止痛錠劑治療背痛。」

3) 如果你對正在進行的程序不清楚，可以請醫師或護士再慢慢解釋一遍。

☞ For example: "Excuse me, could you please explain that again?"

例如：「對不起，可不可以請你再解釋一遍？」

4) 確定你非常清楚吃藥必需注意的事項和每次服用的劑量。複述用藥說明，必要的話，把它寫下來。

☞ For example: "Take one tablet by mouth every morning."

例如：「每天早上口服一個藥片。」

5) 回答問題時使用簡單、易懂的句子。

☞ For example: "Yes, I did." "No, I haven't." "I don't know."

例如：「是，我有。」、「不，我沒有。」、「我不知道。」

A⁺系列 英文從C躍升到A⁺的輕鬆學習！

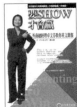

要SHOW才會贏－外商總經理卓文芬教你英文簡報

1書1DVD 定價：280元

從補習班名師到AIG友邦信用卡總經理，英文程度、簡報功力、職場嗅覺、業務能力一把罩，更重要的是，她深諳「要Show才會贏」的工作哲學。

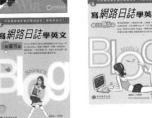

寫網路日誌學英文－辦公室熟女篇

1書1CD 定價240元

- 藉Molly的30篇網路日誌，輕鬆學慣用語和句法
- 教你獨創自己的網路日誌風格，秀出個人特色
- 單元句型佐以貼心圖示，情境造句強化組織能力

寫網路日誌學英文－上網獵男篇

1書1CD 定價240元

- 劇中女主角Shiraz穿越網路時空，尋覓Mr. Right的全紀實
- 用最savvy的英文，淋漓盡致表達喜怒哀樂
- 上網交友安全法則，劈腿男、老色鬼、歐吉桑Bye－bye

英文單字就在我身邊

作者：黑川裕一　定價200元

- 由「我」出發聯想式記憶，速學熟記日常最好用的1200個英文單字
- 15個由「我」為出發的字彙類別，「家人、同事、朋友」讓單字與「自我」產生關連
- 97款有趣練習，「大頭貼記憶、心理測驗」量身定作你的生活寫真

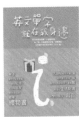

十五分鐘英文早操－用電影對白學公開演說

作者：Jeff Hammons　1書1CD，定價：250元

- 56部經典電影精選對白：美麗境界、顛慄空間、海底總動員、槍上富家女...等
- 28個生活情境主題：自我介紹、公布事情、鼓舞士氣、派對時光...等
- 內容有趣：精選題材經典對白，說說更生動
- 主題豐富：演說對談精妙絕倫，讓您隨學即用

十五分鐘英文早操－用電影對白學私人對談

作者：Jeff Hammons　1書1CD，定價：250元

- 56部經典電影精選對白：史瑞克、紅磨坊、鐵達尼號、征服情海...等
- 28個生活情境主題：情人之間、朋友之間、家人之間、金錢問題...等
- 招式易學：依葫蘆畫葫蘆，在練習中培養語感
- 互動學習：多樣主題單元，跟述朗讀皆上口

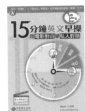
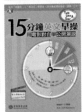

國家圖書館出版品預行編目資料

醫病診療 900 句典 / Lily Yang 作；林曉芳譯.
——初版.——臺北市：貝塔，2007〔民 96〕
　面：　　公分

ISBN 978-957-729-625-2（平裝附光碟片）

1. 醫學英語—會話

805.188　　　　　　　　　　　　95026313

醫病診療 900 句典

Overheard in the Hospital

作　　　者 / Lily Yang
總 編 審 / 王復國
譯　　　者 / 林曉芳
執 行 編 輯 / 杜文田

出　　　版 / 貝塔出版有限公司
地　　　址 / 台北市 100 館前路 12 號 11 樓
電　　　話 / (02)2314-2525
傳　　　真 / (02)2312-3535
郵　　　撥 / 19493777 貝塔出版有限公司
客服專線 / (02)2314-3535
客服信箱 / btservice@betamedia.com.tw

總 經 銷 / 時報文化出版企業股份有限公司
地　　　址 / 桃園縣龜山鄉萬壽路二段 351 號
電　　　話 / (02) 2306-6842

出版日期 / 2014 年 6 月初版五刷
定　　　價 / 250 元
I S B N：978-957-729-625-2

Overheard in the Hospital by Lily Yang
Copyright 2007 by Beta Multimedia Publishing
Published by Beta Multimedia Publishing

貝塔網址：www.betamedia.com.tw

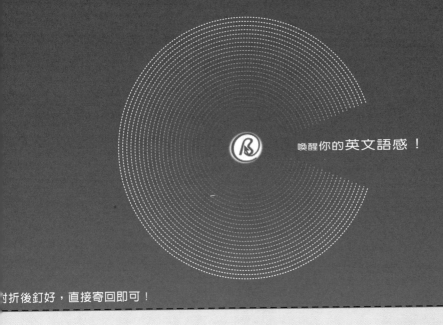

喚醒你的英文語感！

對折後釘好，直接寄回即可！

廣　告　回　信
北區郵政管理局登記證
北台字第14256號
免　貼　郵　票

100 台北市中正區館前路12號11樓

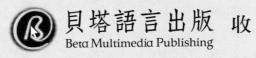

貝塔語言出版 收
Beta Multimedia Publishing

寄件者住址 □□□

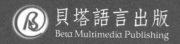

貝塔語言出版
Beta Multimedia Publishing

讀者服務專線（02）2314-3535　讀者服務傳真（02）2312-3535
客戶服務信箱 btservice@betamedia.com.tw
www.betamedia.com.tw

謝謝您購買本書！！

貝塔語言擁有最優良之英文學習書籍，為提供您最佳的英語學習資訊，您填妥此表後寄回（免貼郵票）將可不定期免費收到本公司最新發行書訊及活動訊息！

姓名：＿＿＿＿＿＿＿＿＿＿　性別：□男 □女　生日：＿＿＿＿年＿＿＿＿月＿＿＿＿日

電話：(公)＿＿＿＿＿＿＿＿＿＿(宅)＿＿＿＿＿＿＿＿＿＿(手機)＿＿＿＿＿＿＿＿＿＿

電子信箱：＿＿＿＿＿＿＿＿＿＿＿＿＿＿＿＿＿＿＿＿＿＿

學歷：□高中職含以下 □專科 □大學 □研究所含以上

職業：□金融 □服務 □傳播 □製造 □資訊 □軍公教 □出版 □自由 □教育 □學生 □其他

職級：□企業負責人 □高階主管 □中階主管 □職員 □專業人士

1 . 您購買的書籍是？＿＿＿＿＿＿＿＿＿＿＿＿＿＿＿＿＿＿＿＿＿

2 . 您從何處得知本產品？(可複選)

　　□書店 □網路 □書展 □校園活動 □廣告信函 □他人推薦 □新聞報導 □其他

3 . 您覺得本產品價格：

　　□偏高 □合理 □偏低

4 . 請問目前您每週花了多少時間學英語？

　　□不到十分鐘 □十分鐘以上，但不到半小時 □半小時以上，但不到一小時

　　□一小時以上，但不到兩小時 □兩個小時以上 □ 不一定

5 . 通常在選擇語言學習書時，哪些因素是您會考慮的？

　　□ 封面 □內容、實用性 □品牌 □媒體、朋友推薦 □價格 □其他＿＿＿＿＿＿＿＿＿

6 . 市面上您最需要的語言書種類為？

　　□聽力 □閱讀 □文法 □口說 □寫作 □其他＿＿＿＿＿＿＿＿＿＿

7 . 通常您會透過何種方式選購語言學習書籍？

　　□書店門市 □網路書店 □郵購 □直接找出版社 □學校或公司團購

　　□其他＿＿＿＿＿＿＿＿＿＿

8 . 給我們的建議：＿＿＿＿＿＿＿＿＿＿＿＿＿＿＿＿＿＿＿＿＿＿＿＿＿＿＿＿＿

＿＿＿＿＿＿＿＿＿＿＿＿＿＿＿＿＿＿＿＿＿＿＿＿＿＿＿＿＿＿＿＿＿＿＿＿＿＿＿

喚醒你的英文語感！

Get a Feel for English !